Coming Clean

A Guide to Detoxifying the Body for Better Health

by Steven H. Horne

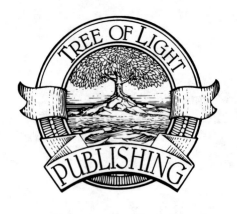

**Tree of Light Publishing
P.O. Box 911239
St. George, UT 84791
800-416-2887**

Table of Contents

Chapter One

Why Cleansing?

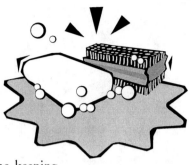

Most people spend a lot of time keeping things clean. We bathe, wash dishes, vacuum our carpets, sweep our floors, take our cars to the car wash, and launder our clothes. However, very few people ever give thought to the idea of internal cleanliness. But, it isn't just the outside of the body and our environment that must be kept clean. We need to be clean on the inside, as well.

Every day the body creates waste products as we consume foods and beverages and burn them for energy. The elimination of these by-products of metabolism is so important that the body has many different systems for breaking them down and expelling them. Were it not for the incredible efficiency of the lymphatic system, the liver, the kidneys, the sweat glands and oil ducts in the skin, the colon, and the mucus membranes of the sinuses and lungs, the body would suffocate in its own waste in a couple of days.

Just because we aren't dead, however, doesn't mean that our eliminative organs are working at peak efficiency. When a furnace, automobile, or any other mechanical device starts to get dirty, its efficiency diminishes. The same is true for the body. If the efficiency of one or more eliminative channels drops just 10 or 20% it won't be enough to kill us, but it certainly will have a gradual, and cumulative, effect on our energy level and health.

That's why traditional herbalism and naturopathy have always placed a heavy emphasis on hygiene, not just external hygiene, but internal hygiene as well. Therapies dedicated to opening up and strengthening eliminative channels have been collectively known as "cleansing" therapies.

Cleansing is especially important in modern society. While public sanitation and attention to external cleanliness have helped to ensure we don't have plagues or get diarrhea from contaminated water, we have a new problem on our hands—environmental pollution.

Every day we are exposed to hundreds (if not thousands) of chemicals, many of which did not even exist 100 years ago. These chemicals are present in the air we breathe, in the water we drink, in the food we consume and products that come in contact with our skin.

For example, the foods we eat contain traces of agricultural chemicals, pesticides, herbicides and fungicides that are used on crops. Processed foods are also laced with additives—preservatives, artificial flavorings and colorings, emulsifiers, anti-caking agents, texture enhancers and so forth.

We have air pollutants from automobiles and industry. We have water pollutants from agricultural runoff, industrial contamination, and even from the water treatment delivery systems that bring treated water into our homes.

There are also numerous chemicals in our cleaning products, cosmetics, fabrics, furniture and building materials. So many, in fact, that people who move into a new home often experience headaches, aches and pains, lethargy and other symptoms of environmental illness. This happens because of the outgassing of formaldehyde, solvents, and other chemicals found in carpets, paints, glues, wood and other materials used to build the homes.

For instance, I once had an employee who started getting migraines after moving into a new trailer home. When I encouraged her to open all the windows and air the place out for a couple of weeks, and fill her house with plants to purify the air, the headaches stopped.

Of course, we are assured that these chemicals are safe because they've all been tested—right? Well, laying aside the fact that some of these chemicals haven't been properly tested, there is still a problem with the research that has been done. These chemicals are typically tested one at a time to determine safe levels. They aren't tested in combination, but we are exposed to them in combination every day.

The body can handle small amounts of toxins. It does so all the time. Even natural foods have small amounts of toxic materials.

That's why the body is equipped with detoxification systems. These detoxification processes are part of our immune system. So, if we were exposed to these chemicals one at a time, the body could probably handle them, just as the research suggests. The problem is that we're getting small amounts of many different toxins, which, compounded by the problem of nutritional deficiencies caused by consuming refined and processed foods, causes the body's detoxification systems to become overwhelmed.

So, the more we minimize our exposure to toxins, the less stress we place on our immune system. We don't need to be paranoid about toxins. (I've met people who are so obsessed with this issue that they live in constant fear and worry; and that's not good for your health, either.) We just need to use common sense and avoid environmental toxins and chemicals as much as we can. In addition, we can also provide nutrients that will enhance the function of the immune system to help us deal with the toxins we can't avoid.

When it has the nutrition it needs, the body has the capacity to ramp up its efforts to flush toxins. We've all experienced the body's ability to get rid of toxins when we've thrown up after eating tainted food. Perhaps you can also remember a time when your sinuses started to run after you inhaled some smoke or irritating chemicals.

Illnesses That May Involve Environmental Toxins

- Allergies
- Arthritis
- Asthma
- Autism
- Autoimmune Disorders
  - Fibromyalgia
  - MS
  - Lupus
- Birth Defects
- Cardiovascular Disease
- Cancer
- Chronic Headaches
- Fatigue
- Kidney Diseases
- Learning Disabilities
  - ADD/ADHD
  - Mental Retardation
  - Senility
- Liver Disease
- Memory Loss and Senility
- Neurological Disorders
- Obesity
- Skin Disorders
  - Eczema
  - Psoriasis
  - Rashes

In fact, it is likely all chronic illness involves some toxicity!

3

Another example of these defensive mechanisms at work is getting a skin rash after exposure to an irritating substance. All of these defense mechanisms—vomiting, diarrhea, sinus drainage (including sneezing and coughing), and skin eruptions—are demonstrations of the ability of the immune system to throw off an irritating substance.

Unfortunately, most people don't understand this process. They think that the vomiting, diarrhea, nausea, sinus drainage or skin eruption is caused by the disease. So, they go to the doctor or drugstore seeking some medication that will block or halt these efforts of the body to flush irritants. The drugs themselves are also chemicals and add a further burden to the immune and detoxification systems of the body, thus sending the system on a downward spiral. As the body is unable to eliminate the backlog of toxins, they irritate, inflame and damage various tissues and organs.

Inflammation can be thought of as the "mother" of all diseases. Nearly all chronic and degenerative diseases begin with an inflammatory process, including heart disease and cancer. These diseases are the end result of damage from uneliminated toxins and nutritional deficiencies.

When the body can't flush the toxins, it tries to find some way to store or neutralize them in order to protect tissues from further inflammation or damage. Fat deposits, cysts, growths, weakened tissues and organs can all wind up as toxic waste storage facilities. The fact that fats sequester toxins also helps explain why more than 60% of us are overweight. In the end, the weakened organs and tissues where the toxins often wind up are so diseased they have to be surgically removed. (Which, when one thinks about it, could be thought of as a really extreme method of detoxification!)

Fortunately, there is another answer to the diseases caused by these toxins. It's called cleansing, and it's a very simple process. It's easy to do and inexpensive, too. And, while cleansing isn't a "cure-all," you'll probably be amazed at how many of your minor aches and pains, chronic health problems, and even emotional problems diminish or simply disappear when you stop trying to suppress the efforts of the body to eliminate toxins and start helping it.

Chapter Two

The Many Benefits of Fasting

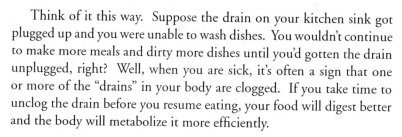

GROAN!

Have you ever noticed that little children and animals tend to shun food when they are sick? There is a reason for this. In most acute illness, the body is congested, and when the body is congested it does little good to put more food into it. It just clogs the system more.

Think of it this way. Suppose the drain on your kitchen sink got plugged up and you were unable to wash dishes. You wouldn't continue to make more meals and dirty more dishes until you'd gotten the drain unplugged, right? Well, when you are sick, it's often a sign that one or more of the "drains" in your body are clogged. If you take time to unclog the drain before you resume eating, your food will digest better and the body will metabolize it more efficiently.

Okay, maybe you're not into the kitchen stuff, so here's another analogy for those of you who are more mechanically inclined. Think of what happens to a car when the air filter is dirty, the oil needs to be changed and the carburetor and spark plugs are getting fouled. The car no longer burns fuel efficiently, which reduces performance. It also increases the amount of "gunk" being generated by the engine, which causes the engine to get even more clogged up. If one takes the time to clean the carburetor, change the oil and replace the spark plugs and filters, the engine will burn cleaner and more efficiently.

Just like an automotive engine or our household plumbing, the body gets "clogged" periodically. When this happens, the body needs a nutritional "lube, oil and filter service" or an herbal "drain opener" to clean it out so that it can run efficiently again.

Of course, I'm not suggesting that cleansing is the only thing we need to keep the body healthy. Obviously, the body also needs exercise, rest and good nutrition. But, the body isn't going to be able

5

to utilize good nutrition properly if it's congested, and you won't feel like exercising when your metabolic "engine" isn't running efficiently. You probably won't sleep very well when the body's drains are plugged, either. So, in most cases, if you want to improve your health, a good place to start is by doing a cleanse.

The most basic of all cleanses is a fast. In fact, fasting is one of the oldest and most effective natural healing techniques. As I mentioned at the beginning of this chapter, it's also instinctive, since small children and animals don't eat when they don't feel well.

"Starving" Illness

Some of us have been taught to "eat to keep up your strength" when we're sick, but this is bad advice. Even though everyone has heard the sage wisdom of the famous Greek physician Hippocrates, "Feed a cold and starve a fever," practically nobody understands what it means. His advice becomes clearer if you render it as "if you feed a cold, you will have to starve a fever." In other words, it's not wise to feed a cold or a fever. Both need to be "starved" out with fasting because these illnesses are signs the body is congested with metabolic waste.

Many modern Western herbalists and naturopaths have discovered the incredible value of "starving" colds, flu, fevers and other acute ailments. So, next time you feel a cold or flu coming on, stop eating and do some cleansing! Putting food into the body when you're ill is like running more water into a sink with a plugged drain—it's just going to make the problem worse.

Of course, while water is not likely to help a plugged kitchen drain, water is exactly what the body needs when its "drains" are clogged. The old adage, "Go to bed, rest and drink plenty of fluids," is probably the best advice ever written as basic therapy for acute illness. Every eliminative channel of the body needs water to function properly. Simply resting and flushing the system with liquids will help you get over most colds, flu, and other minor ailments faster than an OTC (over-the-counter) medication at your local drugstore or supermarket.

Detoxifying in chronic illness isn't much different—it just takes longer. The body has likely burned up a lot of its nutritional reserves in chronic illness, so it probably doesn't have the nutrients it needs to power the detoxification process. That's why one should start slowly and work gradually with chronic illness, even when making dietary changes. Arnold Ehret, a major proponent of fasting and author of *The Mucusless Diet Healing System*, said that most people say, "Here is good food, eat it." He says, "Here is good food, be careful or it will make you feel sick." I experienced this first hand when I was trying to change my diet. I started eating lots of fresh fruits and vegetables, avoided all junk food, and used only whole grains. Within a few days my sinuses were draining copiously, and I remember thinking, "Why is all this good food making me sick?"

It wasn't. It was simply providing a lot of antioxidants, vitamins, minerals and other nutrients to my starving body, which was allowing my body to initiate some major detoxification. Later, after I learned how to cleanse my body, I was able to eat good food without having these reactions. In fact, after doing a three-month colon cleanse, I was able to eat nothing but cherries for three days and experienced no ill effects. I learned from this that cherries and other fresh fruits can't give you diarrhea, but they can "clean you out" if you are toxic. So, when you're suffering from any kind of chronic illness, it will help to do an herbal cleanse before trying any kind of fasting.

A 24-hour fast once per month is a good basic health-building practice. Periodically, longer fasts can be utilized. For most people, a three- day fast is sufficient, but people have fasted for as long as 40 days. I've done a water fast for five days, but I'm not recommending long fasts like that for health purposes, here.

Juice Fasting

People who are hypoglycemic, that is, they suffer from low blood sugar, have a hard time fasting. If you're one of these people, it's

Contraindications for Fasting and Cleansing

Fasting is not advisable for small children, pregnant and nursing mothers and severely weak and debilitated persons. The same restrictions for apply to cleansing in geneeral. In severe chronic and degenerative diseases cleansing should be undertaken under professional supervision. If in doubt, consult a holistic physician or a naturopath for advice.

probably better to do a juice fast. It's also better to do a juice fast if you're going to fast for more than 24 hours. A juice fast involves abstaining from solid food, and drinking some kind of fresh fruit or vegetable juice whenever you feel hungry. Plenty of water should also be consumed while on a juice fast.

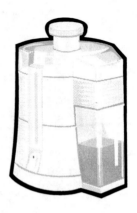

I've done many juice fasts, usually for a period of two or three days. I also fast on water or juice for short periods 4-12 hours when I'm feeling congested, bloated, constipated, and "foggy" in the head. As soon as the body clears itself, these symptoms disappear and I'm able to go back to eating regular food again.

I've also successfully used juice fasting with family and friends. My mother cured herself of rheumatoid arthritis using juice fasting, based on the recommendations of nutritionist Paavo Airola in his book, *There is a Cure for Arthritis*. She had an attack of this disease that left one of her arms virtually paralyzed. It was so bad she was wearing a sling to hold her arm. After I gave my mother Dr. Airola's book, she bought a juicer and started doing regular juice fasts. In combination with some colon cleansing and some anti-inflammatory herbal remedies like Joint Support, Yucca and Devil's Claw, my mother's arthritis cleared up within a month. The famous herbalist Dr. John Christopher also described this type of juice fast cleansing in his booklet, *Dr. Christopher's Three-Day Cleansing Program*.

I helped a close friend of mine overcome diabetes by doing juice fasting with vegetable juices to stabilize her blood sugar levels. She was so "whacked out" from the blood sugar imbalances that she was having a hard time thinking straight. Since she was a neighbor, I had her come to my house every day and we made the juices from vegetables like carrots, beets and celery and I sent her home with that day's supply. In combination with some blood sugar balancing herbs like licorice and goldenseal, she was able to get completely off her blood sugar medication and cured herself of Type II diabetes. (Although her doctor told her that she couldn't claim she cured herself of diabetes since it is an "incurable" condition!)

These are just a few examples from my own personal experience. There are many books that tell similar stories of how people have used fasting and juice fasting to help themselves heal from many chronic health problems.

When juice fasting, it's important to have a supply of fresh, raw juice. This means one will either need to own a juicer, or have a source to buy fresh, unpasteurized juice. It is best to stick with one type of juice for the duration of the fast. Raw unfiltered apple juice is a good choice because it has a mild laxative action. However, if one has blood sugar issues it should be diluted half and half with water, or the person should opt to use vegetable juices, as they don't raise blood sugar levels as much. '

One of the easiest (and most effective) juice fasts is to fast using lemon water sweetened with real maple syrup. I prefer grade B maple syrup when I can find it because it is darker and has a higher mineral content than grade A maple syrup, which is more sugary. However, I've used both. You can make the lemon drink anyway you want, but I like to use about 4 lemons in a half gallon of water and then sweeten with maple syrup to taste. This is drunk throughout the day.

Lemon is great because it helps both the liver and the kidneys flush toxins. It is particularly helpful for flushing waste acids from the body. In my most recent experiences with this program, I've been adding Thai-Go to the lemon water. This makes a very tasty drink, and adds a lot of anti-inflammatory and antioxidant power to the drink. If you're interested in learning more about this cleanse, read *The Master*

Supplements to Help Hypoglycemics With Fasting

People with low blood sugar often have a difficult time fasting. Doing a vegetable-juice fast will help. However, if you find that fasting causes headaches, dizziness, weakness, extreme hunger, etc., you may need to take something to help balance your blood sugar while fasting. Licorice root is very good for this. Take 2 capsules three times daily. Super Algae or spirulina are other good choices. They can be taken alone (2-4 capsules 2-3 times per day) or along with licorice root. Super Algae and spirulina supply protein which keeps blood sugar levels stable.

Cleanser, by Stanley Burroughs, which explains how to do this type of juice fasting.

The 24- hour fast or a two or three day juice fast once a month can have many health benefits. First, it eliminates allergy-causing foods from the diet, which results in the elimination of allergy-induced health symptoms. Juice fasting can help reduce chronic pain, relieve digestive upset, clear thought processes, create stronger resistance to disease and increase energy.

A fast should always be broken by eating a meal of fresh fruits or vegetables. Never "pig out" when breaking a fast! Eat light at first and gradually reintroduce heavier foods.

Of course, you don't need to fast in order to do a cleanse, but there are some advantages to combining fasting with cleansing. First of all, it accelerates the detoxification process, making any herbal cleansing program more effective. This is because you aren't taking any food allergens or additives into the body, so all your body's detoxification mechanisms are concentrating their efforts on getting rid of old toxins. Second, because you aren't taking any food allergens or toxins into the body you get to experience what it feels like to be free of these substances which are dragging down your energy. This makes it easier to identify and avoid foods that are taking away from your health. Most people have no idea what it feels like to be truly healthy because their bodies are so burdened with toxins they think that state is "normal."

Of course, if you can't fast, you can simply try "fasting" from something you know isn't good for you. For example, I sometimes ask clients if they can "fast" from coffee or sugar or dairy products for a week or two. This allows the system to clear itself of the substance and allows them to see how it feels not to be consuming it. Often, when they resume consuming the offending substance, they immediately notice a decline in their health.

In conclusion, there are many ways to use fasting to cleanse the body and improve health. Best of all, fasting doesn't cost you a dime. In fact, you get to save money and improve your health at the same time! Of course, fasting will work even better if we also do things to help open up specific channels of elimination. The chapters that follow will explain how this is done.

Chapter Three

The Body's "Chimneys"

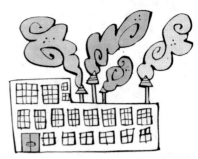

Any system that burns fuel to create energy will produce waste (smoke, ashes, etc.). Because of this, any power plant or engine, from a wood-burning stove to a nuclear reactor, needs periodic cleaning to run efficiently. Furthermore, if that power plant is burning poor quality fuel, or fuel that is laced with contaminants, the system will need to be cleaned more frequently.

The body is a metabolic power plant that produces its own "smoke and ashes." If we don't periodically cleanse the body through fasting and other cleansing procedures, it will initiate its own "self-cleaning cycle." When this happens, we'll think we are sick, because the symptoms generated by the immune system to clean the body out (fever, runny noses, coughing, nausea and diarrhea) are associated with acute illnesses like colds and flu. Unfortunately, most people don't understand this self-cleaning process and seek to "turn it off," or suppress it, rather than support or assist it.

Of course, we've all been taught that "germs" cause these symptoms, but this isn't true. Germs are often involved, but the symptoms themselves are generated by the immune system, not by the germs. The immune system is seeking to expel the germs and the toxins they produce. A toxic body is also a better breading ground for germs, because germs are scavengers which "clean up" dead and diseased material. So, the more toxic the internal environment, the better the environment is for viruses, bacteria, yeast or parasites.

You can think of it like this. Do flies create garbage piles? Of course not, but flies are attracted to garbage piles because they are scavengers in nature which break down garbage. Germs do the same thing in the body.

In fact, it may be possible that the infections we periodically experience are actually part of a detoxification process. These microbes are breaking down the garbage in the body so it can be more easily eliminated. Whether that's true or not, the fact remains that a clean, well-nourished body is very resistant to diseases of all kinds. I've seen this for myself, because when my body has been clean from cleansing and a good diet, I've been able to nurse everyone in my family back to health without getting sick myself.

To understand how we can help the body detoxify instead of trying to suppress its efforts, we need to understand the body's waste removal systems and how they work. We also need to understand the symptoms we experience when these same eliminative channels are overwhelmed or not working. Knowing this helps us choose the right supplements and procedures to support the detoxification systems that are overloaded..

For starters, there are four main systems through which the body can "vent" waste material. They are the mucus membranes of the respiratory tract, the intestinal tract, the urinary tract and the skin. Women have an extra "chimney" because they can also eliminate waste via the menstrual cycle.

In addition to these main waste-removing channels, there are also two internal detoxification systems. The liver is capable of performing many biochemical processes that break toxic compounds down into simpler components, while the lymphatics carry waste material away from tissues.

In addition, each cell also has mechanisms for detoxification that need to be supported. These cellullar detoxification systems use enzymes and nutrients like antioxidants to process toxins.

Let's take a brief look at each of these eliminative systems of the body and what happens when it gets clogged.

The Intestines

For most North Americans, the first channel of elimination to become sluggish is the colon. People who have studied the "hunter-gatherer" peoples, who lived off the land, have observed that they had one bowel movement for every meal they ate. This is because of the

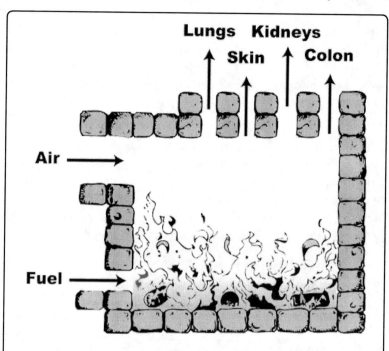

Lungs Kidneys
Skin Colon

Air

Fuel

The Body Furnace

This model is one I've used for years to help people understand how the body works. It suggests that the body is like a wood burning stove, which takes in fuel and air, burns it to create heat and energy, and then vents off the waste.

It also illustrates the idea that the body has four main "chimneys" or eliminative systems. When one or more of these eliminative systems is clogged, the others help take up the slack. So, if the colon is plugged, we might get a lot of sinus drainage or develop skin problems as these systems take over the burden of eliminating the excess waste.

Unfortunately, when most people experience this "toxic overload" and one of these systems is "venting" the excess waste, they think they are "sick." So they seek out some suppressive medication to halt the symptom. This is like putting a "cork" into one of the chimneys. The drugs they are taking relieve the symptoms, but simply congest the body further, putting it on a downward spiral of failing health.

Cleansing is simply the process of being a "chimney sweep"— opening and clearing the body's eliminative systems.

high amount of fiber they had in their diet. These people were free of all types of bowel problems such as diverticulitis, hemorrhoids, colitis, irritable bowel syndrome, constipation and even colon cancer. They were also robust and generally healthy, having a strong resistance to infectious disease.

Dr. Henry G. Bieler spent many years healing patients with food. In his book, *Food Is Your Best Medicine*, Dr. Bieler describes how toxemia in the colon eventually produces symptoms of disease in other parts of the body. He calls the lining of the digestive tract the first line of immune defense. The mucous membranes that line our intestines are not only designed to absorb nutrients, but to reject poisonous substances and waste. They act as a type of selective filter.

When these membranes are overloaded with toxic material, they become irritated and inflamed. They no longer are able to process nutrients correctly and absorb them properly. This gives rise to colitis and other inflammatory bowel disorders, including Crohn's disease, celiac disease and ulcerative colitis. All of these diseases involve a breakdown of the intestinal mucosa due to inflammatory processes.

Inflammation and swelling in the intestines also lead to an increased absorption of toxic materials into the blood and lymph streams, a condition known as leaky gut syndrome. This gut leakage creates a cascade of negative reactions that adversely affect every system of the body.

Modern medical research is confirming that there are links between intestinal problems and chronic illness. Research has linked a wide variety of health problems with intestinal inflammation. These include arthritis, allergies, eczema and other skin diseases, asthma and even some cancers.

The experience of myself and other natural healers is that problems with the intestinal mucosa are also linked to colds, fevers, chronic sinus problems, earaches, sore throats, swollen lymph nodes, body odor, acne, urinary tract infections, headaches, muscle stiffness and weight gain.

Research is also proving that there is a basis for "gut instincts." Science has shown that there are complex networks of nerves and neurotransmitters in our intestines and that they communicate vital information to our brain. This is why science has been able to link intestinal inflammation with "mental" diseases like depression, ADHD and schizophrenia.

The path from the brain to the gut also plays a strong role in the development of inflammatory bowel disorders. Strong emotions and stress responses are well-known triggers of intestinal "dis-stress."

Liver

The liver is the back-up system to the intestines. All of the blood coming out of the intestinal tract passes through the liver via the hepatic vein before being carried to other parts of the body. 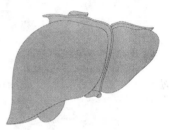 Just as the intestines are the primary external organ of elimination (meaning the primary way toxins are pushed out of the body), the liver is the most important internal organ of detoxification (meaning it has the job of neutralizing toxins that get into the system).

Dr. Bieler referred to it as the second line of immune defense. When the first line of defense (the intestinal mucosa) has been breached, the liver acts as a backup defensive perimeter to keep toxic substances out of the blood. It is the body's biochemical workhorse because it contains hundreds of enzyme systems that both break down toxins and process nutrients.

In modern society, the liver takes a heavy beating. Not only does it have to process toxins generated by poorly digested nutrients and leaky gut syndrome, it also has to process food additives and environmental toxins. With the average person in North America consuming several pounds of these chemicals each year, the liver has its job cut out for it.

The liver needs nutrients in order to perform its biochemical wizardry. So, when we combine poor nutrition with an excessive burden of toxins, the liver will start to breakdown. This is easily exemplified by what happens when a person consumes too much alcohol. Alcohol is a metabolic poison which impairs many body functions, so when a person consumes alcohol, the liver starts enzymatically converting it to sugar (a nutrient).

The liver can easily handle this process when one drinks in moderation. Excessive drinking, on the other hand, overburdens the liver. The drinker winds up with a hangover. They may get nauseous and throw up. They wake up feeling lethargic and sluggish, and may have a headache, too.

One doesn't need to drink to suffer from these symptoms, which are typical reactions to an overworked liver. Many people wake up with a mild "hung over" feeling. They are lethargic, sluggish, nauseous, dull in the head or suffer from mild morning headaches. I see these as signs that their liver is congested and burdened with toxins.

The reason liver congestion is involved in nausea and vomiting is because the liver uses the gallbladder as an organ of elimination. The liver will always try to neutralize toxins, but when faced with an excessive load, it will send them back to the intestinal tract via the gallbladder. This causes the bile to be irritating, so the small intestines want to get this irritation out of the body via the shortest possible route, which happens to be up, not down.

Nausea is the feeling we get when the intestines start trying to push something up into the stomach, instead of down towards the colon. It is caused by a reversal of the normal flow of peristalsis. If this effort is successful, we throw up and the irritants are eliminated. If it is unsuccessful, we experience diarrhea as irritants are flushed out the other direction. Often we get a little of both.

Over time, the liver, lacking essential nutrients and burdened with an excessive load of toxins, starts to weaken. As the liver gets weaker, it becomes less efficient in filtering toxins, and the body's second line of immune defense starts to crumble. This gives rise to frequent headaches, sluggishness, lethargy, skin problems (acne, eczema, etc.), weight gain, stuffy, bloated feelings in the abdomen, high or low cholesterol, abdominal blood fat levels, thyroid problems and PMS symptoms in women.

Kidneys

While the liver's primary job is to prevent toxins from the gastrointestinal tract from entering the blood, the primary job of the kidneys is to filter these wastes out once they are in the blood. So, when the first and second lines of defense have been breached, the kidneys now take a hit from the excessive load of toxins.

When the urinary passages are overwhelmed with irritants they will also become inflamed. This can give rise to various inflammatory disorders of the urinary tract, such as nephritis and urethritis, and problems like burning urination, irritable bladder and frequent kidney and bladder infections. Skin eruptive diseases, swollen lymph nodes, fluid retention and reproductive problems can also be linked to an overburdened urinary system.

Acid is the primary waste material the kidneys filter out of the blood. Acid is the principle by-product of cellular metabolism, i.e., the "smoke" of the metabolic fire inside the cells. As the kidneys weaken from nutritional deficiency and an overload of toxins, they become less efficient at removing acid waste.

When the kidneys can no longer handle the acid load, the body has to adopt other measures to neutralize the acid. It "borrows" potassium and magnesium from muscles and calcium from bones to buffer the acid. This results in a breakdown of structural systems in the body, causing muscle tension and pain, headaches, back pain, leg pain, weakened bones (osteoporosis) and weakened joints (arthritis). The calcium used to buffer these acids can also result in kidney stones and calcification of tissues.

In Chinese medicine, the kidneys were thought to "build the bones," so the Chinese saw the connection between the kidneys and the structural system of the body. This is why they saw the kidney energy as part of the body's foundation. Weak knees, weak ankles, leg pains, back pain, etc. usually suggest a need to strengthen kidney function and balance the pH of the body.

Skin

The skin is the largest organ of elimination and serves as a back-up eliminative channel to both the kidneys and the liver. It's really two organs of elimination in one. The sweat glands have the capacity to take some of the load off the kidneys when there are too many water-soluble toxins in the blood. To do this, the body creates a fever in order to try to force the sweat glands to open up and increase elimination through the skin. People have used this detoxification mechanism as an aide to health and healing by taking saunas or steam baths, sitting in sweat lodges, exercising vigorously or just taking hot baths to induce perspiration. This takes a load off the kidneys by filtering toxins through the skin.

Excessive body odor is a sign that the body is toxic. Toxins eliminated through the sweat glands are broken down by bacteria, creating unpleasant odors. Plugging up the sweat glands, using antiperspirant deodorants, simply congests this eliminative system resulting in a more toxic body.

Rashes are usually the result of an eliminative process through the sweat glands. The rash is usually an inflammation of the skin created by the toxins being eliminated through the skin.

The skin also contains oil ducts, which act as the other eliminative channel in the skin. These oil glands secrete an oily substance onto the skin to keep it soft and moist, but they can also be used as a back up eliminative organ for fat-soluble toxins. Normally, fat-soluble toxins are eliminated from the body by being processed in the liver into water-soluble toxins (which are flushed through the kidneys), or into fatty compounds that are dumped into the bile.

These fatty toxins can also be eliminated through the oil glands in the skin when the liver is congested. When oil ducts have to eliminate toxic fats, they become inflamed. This results in skin problems like pimples, blackheads, and pox (as in chicken pox or small pox). Fat-soluble toxins trapped in the fatty layer underneath the skin will also create itching, and may also cause rashes.

While we're on the subject of the skin, we also need to mention that the hair can be used to eliminate some toxins, especially heavy metals. That is why hair analysis can be used as a method of detecting problems with heavy metal poisoning.

Remember that the skin is not a primary organ of elimination. It is a back up system. So, if there are problems with the skin, one can be assured that there are problems with the colon, liver and/or kidneys. One can assist the eliminative process through the skin, but one also has to take care of the primary organs of elimination to stop the toxins at the source.

Lymphatic System

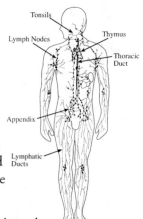

Tonsils

Lymph Nodes

Thymus

Thoracic Duct

Appendix

Lymphatic Ducts

The lymphatic system is the tissue cleansing system of the body. All cells are bathed in lymphatic fluid, which constitutes the internal environment of the body. Fresh, clean, nutrient-laden lymphatic fluid enters the tissues from the blood stream through blood capillaries. Cells absorb oxygen and nutrients from this fluid, then secrete waste back into it.

Some of this lymph fluid is drawn back into the blood stream at the venous end of the capillaries, carrying carbon dioxide, acid and other waste products to be filtered out by the lungs and kidneys. The rest is drawn into lymphatic capillaries where it is taken to lymph nodes, which act like tiny "sewage treatment" plants. There, white blood cells gobble up debris and other detoxification mechanisms "purify" the lymph before returning it to circulation. The lymph ducts empty into the circulatory system at the base of the neck near the thyroid gland, where iodine from that gland can further "treat" this fluid to purify it.

The lymph system has no pump of its own. It is pumped by deep abdominal breathing and body movement. This is why exercise and deep breathing are critical to detoxification. Most people are shallow breathers. Shallow breathing, combined with a sedentary lifestyle, is a sure-fire recipe for tissue toxicity. Lymphatic herbs can help loosen congested lymph fluid so it can move, but only deep breathing and exercise will actually move it. The exercise doesn't have to be strenuous either. Walking, stretching, swimming, or gently bouncing on a mini-trampoline will all move lymph very effectively, cleansing all the tissues of the body in the process.

Keeping the lymph moving is essential to keeping the environment of the tissues themselves clean, and must be considered in any cleansing program. The lymphatic system is also a major part of our immune system, so keeping the lymphatic system working properly wards off illness in general.

Respiratory System

The respiratory system is the primary channel of elimination for carbon dioxide, one of the by-products of metabolism. It can also serve as a backup system of elimination for the lymphatics.

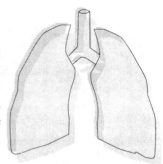

The mucus membranes of the respiratory system secrete a thin protective coating called mucus. This mucus is swept to the back of the throat (from the sinuses) or the top of the throat (from the lungs) where it is either swallowed and excreted through the intestines, or directly expectorated through coughing or spitting. Airborne pollutants will trigger sneezing, coughing and excess drainage as means of flushing pollutants off the surface of the respiratory membranes.

This mucus is composed primarily of lymphatic fluid, so excess mucus can also be created to flush irritants from the lymphatic system. Excess debris from the lymphatic system will be secreted into the bowel if it is clean. If the bowel is impacted and sluggish, however, this lymphatic debris will backup and be secreted through the mucus membranes of the respiratory tract, and possibly through the skin.

So, when the lungs or sinuses are being constantly used as a major channel of elimination, it is because other detoxification systems, particularly the bowels and kidneys, are clogged. So, whenever respiratory congestion is present, look to cleansing the colon and flushing the kidneys as a primary strategy for easing this condition.

Storage of Toxins

When the body is unable to eliminate toxins, it seeks to sequester them. In other words, it tries to round them up and store them somewhere, hopefully in a less vital organ or system. Storing toxins results in cysts, boils, abscesses, growths, tissue deterioration and weight gain. You read that right, excess body fat is often the result of toxins, because fat is one of the body's favorite ways to store toxins.

When a person is chronically ill, their system is always storing a lot of toxins. That's why in all chronic illness, the cleansing process must be done gradually. One doesn't want to release all these toxins out of the tissues and into the blood and lymph all at once. This would simply overwhelm the eliminative organs, causing the person to feel ill. Dizziness, headaches, swollen lymph nodes, fluid retention, sluggishness, fatigue, lethargy and other vague symptoms of malaise are often indications that toxins are in the blood and lymph and are overwhelming the eliminative organs.

So, in chronic illness, one has to gradually open up the eliminative channels. However, just opening the eliminative organs alone isn't going be enough to get rid of stored toxins. One must also activate cellular cleansing mechanisms in the body, because toxins are now trapped inside of tissues and cells. These cells need nutrients such as antioxidants, vitamins, minerals, and enzymes to kick toxins out of the cell and into the lymph. The lymphatics have to be activated to carry these toxins to the bloodstream and the eliminative organs.

Sometimes, when a person who has been chronically ill starts getting better nutrition into the body, they will experience a "healing crisis." Tissues will release toxins and the body will open up various channels of elimination to get rid of them through nausea and vomiting, diarrhea, skin eruptions, sinus drainage or urination. When this happens, the person should fast as discussed in Chapter Two and allow the toxins to be flushed from the system. Support the eliminative processes using the cleansing techniques discussed in this book, rather than suppressing them and driving the toxins back into the tissues.

Putting it All Together

In summary, the body doesn't have just one method of elimination, so when one channel cannot handle all the waste in the body, then another eliminative system will take up the slack. I call this process emergency evacuation. It has also been called vicarious elimination. (See "The Body Furnace" on page 13.)

This emergency evacuation of toxins produces most of the symptoms of acute ailments. When this elimination of excess waste occurs through the digestive tract we call it nausea, vomiting and diarrhea. When it occurs through the urinary system it may produce frequent or burning urination or other signs of kidney or bladder distress. When it occurs through the skin we have body odor, excess perspiration, pimples, acne, rashes, hives and pox. When it occurs through the sinuses and lungs we have bad breath, sinus drainage, runny noses, coughs and other forms of respiratory congestion.

Suppressing symptoms can be likened to putting a "cork" in one or more of the body's "chimneys." This gives the appearance of a cure by eliminating the effect of the disease, but it does not eliminate the cause. In fact, it actually contributes to the underlying cause of disease. Furthermore, when toxins can't be eliminated, they are stored, which gives rise to chronic diseases. Therefore, cleansing should be a primary consideration in all chronic diseases.

The most difficult concept one needs to grasp if one is going to become effective in understanding natural healing is to recognize that we do not want to suppress symptoms of elimination. We want to learn to work with the body, not against it, which means that sometimes we will deliberately make the symptoms worse for a short period of time in order to help the body flush what is irritating it. Once the body has flushed the irritation (toxins), the sense of disease will pass and our health will rapidly return to normal.

In the chapters that follow, we'll learn numerous techniques for supporting the various "chimneys" our body has for eliminating waste. In the next chapter, we'll cover the body's biggest, and most important, chimney—the colon.

Chapter Four

First Things First

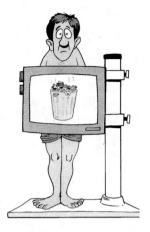

When a little child "needs to go," many a parent has asked the question "Number one or number two?" referring respectively, of course, to the need to empty the urinary tract (#1) or the colon (#2). Well, when it comes to cleansing, these numbers need to be reversed. Unless there is a problem with renal failure, the colon is the primary organ people need to cleanse, which is why number two is number one in detoxification.

At one time people, understood the importance of being "regular" and the problems associated with being "irregular." Today, the importance of regular bowel eliminations, is largely ignored by common people and medical folks alike. However, being "regular" with bowel elimination is essential to health.

Although the colon is sometimes thought of as the body's sewer system, this really isn't true. The colon isn't just an organ of elimination, it's also an organ of assimilation. Here water and electrolytes are absorbed, making the material firmer. Certain minerals and B vitamins, especially B-12 are absorbed here, too. Some nutrients may even be manufactured for our use by the action of friendly bacteria living there.

Whether we want to maintain or regain our health, the gastrointestinal (GI) system is central to our efforts. Our "guts" are equivalent to a plant's roots. It is in our intestines where we interact most intimately with our environment—where we literally transform materials from our environment into us! As the source of water and nourishment and our primary channel of elimination, they constitute our first line of defense against disease. In fact, sixty percent of our immune response is in our GI tract. It's easy to see how dysfunction of the digestive and intestinal system can be linked with so many chronic and degenerative diseases.

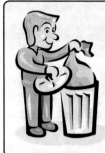

The Importance of Staying "Regular"

Not being regular is like having the local trash man show up on a sporadic, infrequent schedule to pickup your household garbage. Having a house full of smelly trash because the trash man failed to show up isn't very healthy, but that's pretty much what it's like in the body when the colon fails to eliminate properly on a regular basis.

When the small intestine becomes inflamed, we are no longer able to process nutrients and absorb them properly. This gives rise to colitis and other inflammatory bowel disorders, including Crohn's disease, celiac disease, and ulcerative colitis. All of these diseases involve a breakdown of the intestinal mucosa due to inflammatory processes.

Inflammation and swelling in the intestines lead to an increased absorption of toxic materials into the blood and lymph streams, a condition known as leaky gut syndrome. This gut leakage creates a cascade of negative reactions that adversely affect every system of the body. But what causes this intestinal inflammation in the first place?

Factors Which Damage Colon Health

Here are some of the major "enemies" that breach vital lines of defense by causing intestinal inflammation and leaky gut syndrome.

Antibiotics

The intestines contain several pounds of friendly microorganisms that live in a symbiotic relationship with the body. Antibiotics upset the balance of these microbes and increase the risk of inflammation and gut leakage by promoting yeast overgrowth. Yeast exudes an aldehyde secretion that causes swelling (inflammation) in the lining of the small intestine.

Food Allergies

Each of us has our own unique genetic signature, which makes some foods compatible with our body chemistry and other foods incompatible. Food allergies are very common and, although they are difficult to diagnose medically, you can learn to identify foods that cause digestive upset in your body and eliminate them simply by becoming more aware of how foods affect you.

Common food allergens include dairy foods and grains containing gluten (wheat and many other grains, but not buckwheat). Other common food allergens include eggs, legumes (especially soy and peanuts) and nuts. A good place to start is to learn your blood type and avoid foods that are incompatible with it. Tree of Light Publishing (www.treelite.com) produces easy-to-use *Blood Type, pH and Nutrition* charts to help you.

Drugs and Other Chemicals

Anti-inflammatory drugs like ibuprofen have been shown to cause leakiness in the guts. Heavy metal toxicity, smoking, birth control pills and antacids can lead to a build-up of homocysteine, which causes intestinal inflammation. Other chemicals that can upset the balance of our friendly flora and increase intestinal irritation include nitrates, MSG and chlorinated water.

Microorganisms

H. pylori bacteria can trigger food allergies through the leakiness they create in the guts. Toxins from other harmful microbes can also damage and inflame intestinal membranes, such as the yeast mentioned previously. Parasites may also contribute to this problem.

When one understands the information above, one can see that intestinal cleansing isn't just about getting the bowels to move. It's about eliminating sources of irritation which are causing intestinal inflammation and leaky gut syndrome. It's also about rebuilding the integrity of the intestinal mucosa and restoring a proper balance to the friendly flora which live in the intestines. Digestive function also plays a critical role in this process.

Assessing Colon Health

Years ago, I remember how shocked I was when some seasoned natural healers started a discussion about optimal bowel movements at a formal dinner during a Nature's Sunshine convention. Since that time, I've become comfortable with the subject of bowel movements and, while I don't recommend this as a subject for dinner conversation, learning to take note of the shape, type and frequency of your bowel elimination will help you monitor your progress with your health. In the movie, *The Last Emperor*, the Chinese doctors were regulating the young Emperor's diet by examining his stool. You can do the same thing, but first, you need to know what an optimally healthy elimination should look like.

Frequency and Ease of Movements

For starters, most healthy infants (and wild animals) have one bowel movement for each meal they eat. Since most North Americans eat three meals per day, this would translate into three eliminations per day. So, if you have one bowel movement per day (or less) and you eat three meals per day, you're constipated.

Next, your stool should not be difficult to eliminate. You should be able to feel the urge to go, sit down and have the elimination come out in a smooth move. If you have to strain to eliminate, you're constipated.

Shape and Consistency

The shape of the stool is also important. Your colon is a long narrow tube, and the stool should come out in long, narrow pieces. Usually, healthy stools will be banana- or s-shaped, or shaped like a thick piece of rope. If the stool comes out in hard, dry balls, you are constipated and probably dehydrated, too. You are probably lacking in dietary fiber, as well.

The stool should be about the combined thickness of your pointer and middle fingers. If it is larger than this, then you are getting ballooning in the colon, a sign that the colon is lacking muscle tone, and a good colon cleanse is probably in order.

The consistency of the stool tells a lot about what is happening in the digestive tract. The stool should have form, but the form should be loose and probably break up a little on flushing. It should not be thick and fudgy (like peanut butter). If it is, you may not have enough fiber in your diet, or you may have an imbalance in the friendly microbes in the colon.

If the stool doesn't have form and is watery, then you've got diarrhea. When I first tried taking All Cell Detox many years ago (when it was

Normal Doesn't Mean Healthy

Most North Americans think they are regular when they have one movement per day. Although this is "average" for Americans and therefore considered "normal" by just about everyone, including medical doctors, let us remember that the average American is not very healthy. If we want exceptional health, we need to look for what is "natural" and optimal and not necessarily what is average or considered "normal." Optimal colon function is one bowel movement for each major meal we eat.

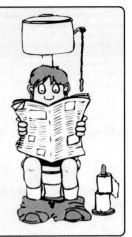

known as Special Formula #1) I thought I was getting diarrhea because I was having three and four bowel eliminations each day. Many of my clients think the same thing when they start taking cleansing herbs. But, if the stool has form, it's not diarrhea. You are just eliminating a backlog of waste.

When there is a watery, unformed stool, the diarrhea can usually be remedied by dietary fiber or activated charcoal. Diarrhea is a sign of acute or chronic intestinal inflammation, which is due to the presence of toxins in the digestive tract (which may be the result of infection or parasites). The fiber absorbs the toxins, but there may also be a need for anti-inflammatory agents, anti-microbial agents or a parasite cleanse. (See Chapter Eight for more information on infections and parasites.) Chronic diarrhea is often a sign of inflammatory bowel disorders and should be checked out by a doctor.

Digestive Function

The stool can also tell you how well your digestive tract is working. If there are undigested food particles in the stool, then you need to work on digestion. Are you chewing your food thoroughly? Do you have sufficient hydrochloric acid and digestive enzymes to break food down properly? If not, Proactazyme or Food Digestive Enzymes may help.

Stools should not float, either. If stools have a greasy sheen and bob around in the toilet like a cork (which makes them very difficult to flush) then you aren't digesting fats properly. Your gall bladder may not be functioning properly to emulsify fats (make them water soluble) for absorption or you may be deficient in lipase enzymes. Try taking Hi-Lipase with meals. Fat Grabbers may also be helpful.

Which also brings us to the subject of stool color. Bile is a major contributor to the color of one's stool. Healthy bile is a yellow color and colors the stool a light brown. When bile is toxic it becomes green or dark green, which makes the stool darker in color. Dark brown or blackish colored stools can be a sign the body is dumping toxins from the liver through the bile, particularly if the stool has a strong odor. If the stool is clay-colored (very light), then the gallbladder may be obstructed or the liver is failing to produce sufficient bile. In either case, support for the liver and gallbladder may be needed. (See Chapter Nine for information on how to help the liver and gallbladder.)

Colon Transit Time

Of course, specific foods, such as chlorophyll and red beets, will also affect stool color. One can use the coloring effect of these foods to determine one's colon transit time. Transit time is the time it takes for waste material from the food we eat to exit the body. Optimally, the body should eliminate any waste material from our food within 18-24 hours of consuming it. Most North Americans have a colon transit time of 72 hours or more, which means the waste material sits in the intestines too long.

To see what your colon transit time is, try eating some red beets and see how long it takes for the red color of the beets to show up in the stool. Also, see how long it takes before no more red color appears in the stool. If the red color shows up and disappears within 24 hours, you're in good shape. If it takes longer, you have a slow colon transit time—a good indication of the need for a colon cleanse. (See Chapters Five and Six.)

If you have red in your stool and haven't been eating beets, you probably have bleeding in the colon or rectum. See a doctor at once to find out what is happening.

Odor

Okay, we all know that waste material is supposed to smell, but it isn't supposed to smell that bad! I'm not suggesting that the stool is supposed to smell sweet, it just isn't supposed to smell rotten.

If the stool has a really foul odor, then something is rotten, and it's not in Denmark, it's inside of you! Foul belching, gas or stool odor is a sign that food is decomposing in your digestive tract. Foods residues are supposed to be eliminated before they start to decompose not after. If the food is decomposing inside of you, then you're absorbing all of that toxic material released from the decomposition process; and that's not a pleasant thought, is it? I assure you that it's not good for your health, either.

Proteins are usually the worst offenders when it comes to creating foul odors—ever smell a rotten egg or piece of fish? So, foul odors are usually a sign that you're not digesting proteins properly. Hydrochloric acid or enzyme supplements (like Protein Digestive Aid, High Potency Protease or Food Digestive Enzymes) will be helpful in breaking down proteins properly. However, general poor digestion and elimination, as well as toxicity will contribute to foul odors. The Chinese Anti-Gas Formula is a good combination to take to reduce gas and odors by improving digestion and elimination. Liquid Chlorophyll is a good supplement to take to reduce odors caused by cleansing programs.

In the next chapter, we'll learn about the basic cleansing tools we can use to detoxify the colon and return it to optimal health. However, it is important to stress again that if you are bleeding from the colon, suffering from chronic diarrhea or have other persistent colon problems, get a medical checkup and find out what you are dealing with. Don't assume that colon cleansing is going to automatically solve every problem you have with the intestines. Be informed about what is happening in your body so you can make informed choices about what is best for your health and monitor the health of your colon regularly to help maintain optimal health.

Chapter Five

Cleansing 101

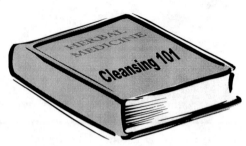

In college, basic classes are always in the 100 series, so a 101 class is one that lays the foundation for more advanced courses a person will take later. For anyone interested in health, understanding how to put together a basic cleansing program should be one of the first subjects they study. So, in our Cleansing 101 course we're going to learn about the components of a basic cleansing program—what they do and why we use them. This will help us evaluate some pre-packaged cleansing programs and learn how to put together our own cleansing program (Chapter Six).

Cleansing herbs are simply herbs that stimulate or strengthen the body's own detoxification systems. The herbs themselves don't really do the cleansing, the tissues do. What the herbs do is supply nutrients that feed and support eliminative functions or they may contain substances that cause an irritation to the tissues, which activates or triggers different detoxification systems.

There are terms used in herbalism that describe the various actions of herbs that strengthen elimination. Herbs that aid bowel elimination fall into two basic categories, *bulk laxatives* (mucilaginous or fiber rich herbs), and *stimulant laxatives* (purgatives and cathartics which irritate the colon, stimulating it to move). There are also two other categories of herbs that will aid bowel elimination—*aperients*, which are very mild-acting laxatives, some of which may actually nourish the colon tissue to gently promote better elimination, and *relaxants* or *antispasmodics*, which can relax bowel spasms which may be causing constipation.

Moving to other eliminative channels, *diuretics* increase the flow of urine through the kidneys, while *lithotriptics* help dissolve kidney stones and calcium deposits. For the lungs and sinuses, *decongestants* and *expectorants* help break up stuck mucus and lymphatic fluid and expel mucus and debris from the respiratory passages. *Blood purifiers* or *alteratives* help to remove toxins from the blood via the liver and lymphatics, while *diaphoretics,* also known as *sudorifics,* increase perspiration through the skin. Elimination through the liver can be aided by *hepatics,* which strengthen liver function, and *chologogues,* which increase the flow of bile. Finally, *lymphatics* and *deobstruents* improve lymphatic flow and remove obstructions from the blood and lymph.

Besides herbs, there are a few non-herbal products that can aid detoxification. *Enzymes* help food digest better, but will also help break toxins down and aid their elimination. *Chelating agents* remove heavy metals and arterial plaque from the body. *Probiotics* are friendly bacteria which improve colon health. *Essential fatty acids* can help the body remove fat-soluble toxins, and *specific nutrients* such as N-Acytl-Cystene, Sam-e, and vitamins and minerals may also aid the process of eliminating specific toxins.

Finally, all cleanses also require *water.* In fact, water is the most critical element needed for any type of cleansing, because all eliminative channels require water to function properly. Water is your primary diuretic, laxative, blood purifier and expectorant. So, while fasting, or on a cleansing program or diet of any kind, it is essential to drink at least 1/2 ounce of water for every pound of body weight per day. So, a 200 pound person needs at least 100 ounces of water each day on a cleanse. Ideally, some type of purified water should be used. I really like using water treated by the Nature's Spring Reverse Osmosis water treatment appliance.

A basic cleanse is usually aimed primarily at the colon, but also requires blood purifiers, chologogues, diuretics, lymphatics and hepatics. These are usually combined in one or more cleansing formulas and taken with water and fiber. If you aren't drinking lots of water and taking some fiber you really aren't going to get a very good cleansing effect. And, as mentioned in the chapter on fasting, the cleanse will also be more effective if it is done while on some type of fast, even if it's just fasting from "junk food."

What follows is a more detailed explanation of the essential elements needed for a basic cleanse.

Fiber

Next to water, fiber is the most important element needed to cleanse the body. Fiber is both a sponge we need to soak up toxins and a scouring pad we need to scrub the colon free of debris. Without adequate fiber, toxins we are releasing from tissues through the action of other cleansing herbs can be reabsorbed and recycled through the

---

Comparing Fiber Blends

Nature's Three is a blend of three fibers—psyllium hulls, apple fiber and oat bran. This makes it a good "broom" for sweeping the colon clean, but it doesn't do much to tonify the colon or deal with the issue of leaky gut syndrome. It's a good choice for serious colon cleansing in situations where there is ballooning in the bowel or a need to clean out bowel pockets (diverticuli).

Psyllium Hulls Combination is a stronger fiber blend, containing psyllium with licorice and hibiscus for flavoring. It is a good fiber for people with ballooning and sluggish bowels.

LOCLO is a blend containing fibers such as psyllium hulls, apple fiber, acacia gum, guar gum, flax seed and oat bran in a base of vegetable powders, broccoli, carrot, red beet, cabbage, Chinese cabbage and tomato. It also contains the herbs rosemary, turmeric and cinnamon. These vegetables and herbs provide an antioxidant effect which reduces intestinal irritation and inflammation. Grapefruit and orange bioflavonoids, hesperidin, citric acid and malic acid have a gentle tonifying action on the mucus membranes of the colon. This is a gentler fiber blend, more suitable for spastic colons and long term use.

Everybody's Fiber is the gentlest of the fiber blends, and the one best suited for irritable bowel, inflammatory bowel disorders, spastic colons and long term use. It contains the gentle fibers of slippery elm, flax seeds, marshmallow and apple pectin. These are combined with herbs which improve digestion, reduce inflammation and tone the bowel to reduce gut "leakiness," including peppermint, fennel, chamomile, uña de gato, and asparagus. Most importantly, Everybody's Fiber contains polysaccharides that act as food for friendly bacteria, which encourages a healthy intestinal flora.

Always take any fiber blend with lots of water.

---

system instead of being eliminated from the body. A blend of fibers is best, which may include fibers such as psyllium hulls, oat bran, apple pectin, slippery elm or flax seed. Nature's Three, Everybody's Fiber, Psyllium Hulls Combination and LOCLO are all good fiber blends for a general cleansing program. See the comparison of these fibers in the sidebar.

If you aren't used to taking fiber, start with a little and work up. Use one heaping teaspoonful in a large glass of water or juice first thing in the morning before breakfast. As the body gets cleaner, the amount of fiber can be increased, up to one heaping tablespoon.

For persons with inflammatory bowel disorders, or cramping of the colon, slippery elm, marshmallow, plantain and other soft fibers and soothing mucilaginous herbs are better choices. Slippery elm is a great choice, but needs to be used in bulk to be really effective. In capsule form, you would have to take 12-24 capsules per day for it to be really effective, which is both expensive and difficult to take. Use a bulk powder, mixed in juice as described above. Since slippery elm doesn't dissolve very readily, you will probably need to use a blender to get the powder to dissolve in liquid. An easier option is to use Everybody's Fiber, a more gentle fiber blend that will dissolve more readily in liquids.

If your stools are really dry, add a little bit of flax seed oil, or freshly ground flax seeds to your fiber drink. Flax is both soothing and lubricating to the colon.

A harsher option, but one that can be very effective, is the use of a fine clay or hydrated bentonite in a cleanse. Clay will draw toxins from bowel tissue and help to remove debris from pockets and ballooned areas in the colon. Clay is not a good option, however, for people with irritable bowel problems, intestinal inflammation, or the tendency to intestinal cramping.

General Cleansing Formulas

In addition to water and fiber, a person needs to take a good cleansing formula, which will stimulate the release of toxins from the tissues. These formulas are usually built around alterative and diuretic herbs, but may also contain hepatics, lymphatics, lithotriptics, laxatives, cholagogues, and even some fiber-rich herbs.

Alteratives, also known as blood purifiers, aid the removal of toxins from the tissues, blood and lymph. They usually help with liver detoxification and may often be cholagogues or hepatics as well. The cholagogue action is important because bile is the way the liver flushes toxins into the digestive tract where the fiber can absorb them. Bile is also nature's natural laxative, as it helps stimulate bowel elimination. Alterative herbs that are also cholagogue, which are often used in cleansing formulas, include burdock, dandelion, yellow dock and milk thistle. Other alteratives include alfalfa, red clover and cleavers.

Diuretics help flush excess fluid from the tissues through the kidneys. This action is important in any cleansing program because the kidneys are the primary means for removing acid waste from the tissues. Diuretics help ensure that the water being consumed on a

Comparing General Cleansing Formulas

Enviro-Detox focuses it's cleansing power on the colon, liver, blood and lymphatics. It contains the alterative or blood purifying herbs burdock, dandelion, red clover, sarsaparilla, echinacea, yellow dock and milk thistle. It also contains fenugreek, ginger and pepsin to improve digestion and help break down toxins in the digestive tract. Marshmallow adds a small amount of soothing fiber, while cascara sagrada gives the formula a mild laxative action. Finally, Enviro-Detox contains friendly bacteria—*Lactobacillus sporogenes*—to help the friendly flora in the bowel.

All Cell Detox has a broader range of cleansing action than Enviro-Detox. While it has some alterative and blood purifying action through black walnut, yellow doc, dandelion and Oregon grape, it also has a strong diuretic effect because it contains goldenseal, parthenium, dandelion and uva ursi. It stimulates digestion through gentian, fenugreek, goldenseal, safflowers, myrrh gum and catnip and reduces intestinal inflammation with goldenseal, myrrh gum and slippery elm. It contains some cascara sagrada for a mild laxative action. It also helps the thyroid because it contains Irish moss and black walnut. All Cell Detox, as it's name implies, is a better formula for general tissue cleansing.

cleanse is used to carry toxins out of the system. Diuretic herbs include juniper berries, buchu, parsley, uva ursi, cornsilk and marshmallow. Some herbs also combine a lymphatic action with a diuretic action, which flushes excess fluid from the tissues and helps drain it out through the kidneys. Herbs that have this action include yarrow, cleavers, red clover and plantain.

Two excellent cleansing formulas are All Cell Detox and Enviro-Detox. Both of these blends have diuretic, laxative, alterative, hepatic, cholagogue and lymphatic actions. The cleansing herb formula should be taken along with the fiber every morning as part of a basic cleansing program. For a more extensive cleanse, take the cleansing formula three times per day.

Enzymes

Unless your diet is 60% raw foods, you need to supplement your diet with extra enzymes. Enzymes help the body break down food efficiently, which results in less intestinal irritation and better absorption of nutrients. They also enhance the immune system and aid cellular detoxification and repair. You will want a plant enzyme supplement that at least contains protease, lipase and amylase. Proactazyme Plus is a good general enzyme supplement. Protease Plus is a protein-digesting enzyme supplement which can be taken to help break down protein material that may be congesting the digestive tract.

Enzymes can also be used as part of a cleansing herbal formula. For example, Small Intestine Detox contains pepsin, a protein-digesting enzyme, in combination with marshmallow, a mucilaginous herb that helps deliver the pepsin to the small intestines where it helps break down proteins. Bowel Detox is a general cleansing formula that includes pancreatic enzymes, pepsin, hydrochloric acid and bile salts to help break down any kind of partially digested food material in the intestines. It also contains fiber and stimulant laxatives. To get the best effect from either of these formulas, they should be taken between meals so that the enzymes and digestive components are used to break down toxins instead of food.

Comparing Enzyme Products for Cleansing

Since much of the toxicity of the digestive tract comes from poorly digested food, it only makes sense to improve digestion with enzymes to increase the effectiveness of cleansing. One can simply take digestive enzymes like Proactazyme, or use a cleansing formula that also contains enzymes. Either way, enzymes will enhance the effectiveness of a cleanse, especially for people with poor digestion.

Small Intestine Detox helps clear mucus and undigested proteins from the small intestines. It contains pepsin, in a base of marshmallow which helps direct the pepsin to the small intestines. It is a good formula for improving nutrient absorption in the small intestines.

Bowel Detox is a broader acting formula, combining enzymes with some general cleansing aids. Its enzyme and digestive enhancing ingredients include HCl, pepsin, pancreatin, bile salts and ginger. It contains several fibers, psyllium hulls, apple pectin, algin (which absorbs heavy metals), bentonite clay, marshmallow, charcoal and kelp. Cascara sagrada supplies a mild laxative action. The vitamins A, C, and E, betacarotene, and the minerals zinc and selenium provide antioxidant and immune-enhancing effects which tone the intestines. Chlorophyll provides a deodorizing effect to the formula, which helps reduce stool odor.

Laxatives

Many people think that cleansing simply involves taking an herbal laxative to stimulate more bowel eliminations. While herbal laxatives may be beneficial in cleansing, they are not always necessary. Often the cleansing formula has a small amount of laxative herbs in it, and combined with the fiber and water, this is enough to keep the bowels moving properly. Laxative herbs include senna, cascara sagrada, turkey rhubarb, butternut bark and buckthorn. Of these, cascara sagrada is one of the most widely used and safest stimulant laxatives. LBS II is a popular and effective stimulant laxative formula, which combines cascara sagrada with hepatics, alteratives, diuretics and herbs that stimulate digestion. For those who have trouble swallowing capsules, the Liquid Cleanse formula is an option. See sidebar for a comparison of these formulas.

Laxatives can be overused, but, if a person is having less than 2-3 bowel movements per day while on a cleanse, then they probably need to include an herbal laxative in any cleanse they do. As an interesting note, cascara sagrada contains a black dye, so, if it is taken regularly for long periods of time (such as year or longer), it will stain the colon black. Many doctors get alarmed when they see this, but there is no evidence that this is causing harm to colon tissue. It also dissipates when use of the cascara is discontinued.

Antimicrobial or antifungal agents

There are two to three pounds of microorganisms in the intestinal tract. Known collectively as "friendly flora," they play a critical role in health, protecting the body against infection, enhancing digestion, and aiding detoxification. When the balance of friendly flora is disrupted, unfriendly microbes such as yeast or harmful bacteria can "take over"

Comparing Stimulant Laxative Formulas

LBS II is a lower bowel formula created by herbalist Stan Malstrom. It is a mild-acting, but effective stimulant laxative formula that contains cascara sagrada, buckthorn, licorice, capsicum, ginger, Oregon grape, turkey rhubarb, couch grass and red clover. In addition to its laxative action, it also has a mild cholagogue and diuretic effect.

The Liquid Cleanse formula contains a blend of aloe vera, red raspberry, senna, cinnamon, fennel, barberry, cornsilk, ginger, dandelion, capsicum, citrus extract and trace minerals. Senna is a stronger laxative, but it's tendency to cause gripping (intestinal spasms) is modified by the other herbs in this formula. Liquid Cleanse also contains herbs that stimulant digestion and have diuretic and hepatic effects.

When a really strong laxative is needed, Senna Combination is the product of choice. Designed for occasional use only, Senna Combination contains senna, fennel, ginger and catnip.

Stimulant laxatives are not recommended for long term use. If you're having trouble eliminating without the use of stimulant laxatives you may have a spastic colon. (See the sidebar on page 41 in the next chapter.)

---

the mix of microbes and cause problems with health. So, it is often necessary to take some kind of antimicrobial or antifungal agent to knock down the bad flora and reestablish the balance of healthy flora. Antifungal herbs include: pau d'arco, garlic and oregano.

Two formulas which can be used to knock down yeast are Yeast/Fungal Detox and Capryllic Acid Combo. Bacteria, such as H. pylori, the organism that causes ulcers, can also be a problem. Gastro Health contains herbs which help destroy H. pylori and other harmful bacteria in the intestines. This topic will be covered in greater detail in Chapters Seven and Eight.

Antiparasitics

Parasites are difficult to diagnose and even medical doctors sometimes miss them. However, if a person has vague health problems that have not been resolved after much effort, one possible cause may be parasites. Some of the symptoms that may point to a possibility of parasites include constant hunger with an unsatisfied appetite, itching rectum, and severe health problems that develop after foreign travel, especially gastrointestinal problems (diarrhea). Antiparasitic herbs include wormwood, tansy, black walnut, butternut bark, and garlic. Parasite cleansing products which make use of these and other antiparasitic herbs include Herbal Pumpkin and Para-Cleanse. If you suspect you might have parasites, you may want to consult a professional herbalist or naturopath for assistance. Parasite cleansing will also be covered in greater detail in Chapter Eight.

Chapter Six

Basic Cleansing Programs

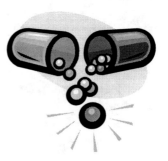

Now that we've mastered our cleansing basics from the previous chapter, we're ready to start assembling some real cleansing programs. We'll start by looking at some pre-packaged cleansing programs and then move to a basic, "do-it-yourself" cleansing program that can be modified to meet individual needs. We'll also give you an enzyme cleansing program and finish with a sample daily cleansing program that can be used regularly to maintain a clean and healthy body.

Pre-Packaged Cleanses

Prepackaged cleanses are convenient and easy to use. Here are three you can choose from. With each, simply take the packets as directed on the label.

Tiao He Cleanse

This cleanse contains a liver formula (Liver Balance), a general cleansing formula (All Cell Detox), a bulking agent (Psyllium Hulls), a stimulant laxative (LBS II), an alterative (Burdock) and an antiparasitic (Black Walnut). It is an excellent basic cleanse, and my personal favorite. It is conveniently packaged and has all the elements needed to do some pretty deep tissue cleansing. The Chinese Liver Balance formula is outstanding at helping the liver to detoxify and All Cell Detox is the best tissue cleansing formula.

There is one weakness to this cleansing program, however. It doesn't have enough fiber to efficiently carry toxins out of the body, so I strongly recommend people using this cleanse add a fiber drink taken first thing in the morning. Also, people need to drink lots of water on this, or any other cleanse.

CleanStart

The CleanStart cleanse comes in two flavors: Apple/Cinnamon and Wild Berry. Its strong point is that it contains a fiber blend that can be mixed with water or juice to absorb toxins. It also contains a stimulant laxative (LBS II) and a general cleansing formula (Enviro-Detox). It is less effective as a deep tissue cleanse, but more effective as a liver and colon cleanse. Again, lots of water should be consumed while on this cleanse.

The only weakness of this cleanse is that the bentonite clay in the fiber drink can be a little harsh for people with inflammatory bowel disorders or a spastic colon. (See sidebar on facing page.) If intestinal gripping or cramping occurs on this cleanse, you need a relaxant or antispasmodic agent such as magnesium or lobelia to counteract the cramping. Also, if you have a very sensitive colon you may be better off doing a custom cleansing program using Everybody's Fiber. Overall, CleanStart is a very simple, but effective, cleansing program.

Dieter's Cleanse

This cleanse was targeted to help people who are seeking to lose weight. It contains both cleansing ingredients and fat-burning ingredients. The cleansing products in this program include a general bowel cleansing formula (Bowel Detox), a general cleansing formula (Enviro-Detox), and a stimulant laxative (LBS II). The ingredients designed to help the body break down fat include a general glandular tonic (Master Gland Formula), an alterative formula that helps the liver with fat metabolism (SF), and the mineral chromium.

The biggest weakness of this cleanse is that it contains almost no fiber except for a small amount in the Bowel Detox formula. So, I again recommend that a person taking this cleanse should add a fiber drink in the morning, and, of course, lots of water.

The above cleansing programs work very well for a majority of people. However, there are special instances where a custom designed cleanse may be preferred.

Basic "Do-It-Yourself" Cleanse

Here's a basic "recipe" for a cleansing program which can be modified according to individual needs.

- 2 capsules of a General Cleansing Formula (All Cell Detox, Enviro-Detox or Bowel Detox) three times daily.

- 2 capsules of Digestive Enzymes (Proactazyme) with each meal. If you have problems with protein-digestion add 1 capsule of High Potency Protease with each meal. If you have problems digesting fats, add 1 capsule of Hi-Lipase with each meal.

- Once per day at breakfast time take one heaping Tablespoon of a fiber blend (Nature's Three, LOCLO or Everybody's Fiber) in a large glass of water or juice. If you have any problems with irritable bowel or inflammatory bowel disorders use Everybody's Fiber and start with 1/2 to 1 teaspoon and slowly work up. If you get constipated, add an herbal laxative formula or magnesium.

- Drink 1/2 ounce of purified water per pound of body weight each day.

Dealing with a Spastic Bowel

Many people have problems with a spastic bowel. When muscles become fatigued, they tend to cramp, and the colon is no exception. When the colon is spastic, bowel movements are sporadic and irregular. Stress will affect bowel the bowel as well.

The continual use of stimulant laxatives like cascara sagrada or LBS II will aggregate a spastic bowel condition. People who can't have bowel movements without using stimulant laxatives usually have a spastic bowel condition. Fruit acids (such as citric, malic and abscrobic acid) and magnesium will help restore normal tone to a spastic bowel.

If you have problems with a spastic bowel, start with 2 Magnesium Complex and 2 Citrus Bioflavionoids with Vitamin C once daily. If the bowels don't start moving normally after 24-48 hours, then increase the dose by 1 Magnesium and 1 Bioflavinoid tablet. Keep increasing the dose every couple of days until the bowel gets loose, then back off the dose. After a few weeks, you should be able to gradually back off the dose.

This cleanse supplies the main items needed in a cleanse. Optionally, you can add the following:

If the bowels move less than 2-3 times daily add:

- 1-3 capsules of an Herbal Laxative (cascara sagrada or LBS II) or one fluid ounce of the Liquid Cleanse formula before bedtime

If griping or intestinal cramping occurs, then add:

- 400-500 mg. of Magnesium (preferably Magnesium Complex) twice daily. You can also try taking 1 capsule of lobelia twice daily or 2 capsules of Cellular Energy three to four times daily. Any of these should help relax bowel spasms.

You can also add antiparasitic, antifungal or antimicrobial agents to this cleanse. (See Chapter Eight for more information on parasites.)

These are only basic suggestions, both the amounts and the products may be varied to account for individual circumstances. This cleanse should be done for a maximum of two to four weeks.

At the end of any cleanse it is a good idea to restore the friendly flora in the digestive tract by taking a round of probiotics. (See Chapter Seven for more information on probiotics.)

The Enzyme Cleanse

I learned about this cleanse from Thomas Easley, a very talented young herbalist. He uses this cleanse as a starting point for people with cancer or other serious chronic ailments. I've tried it, and I really like it because it is very effective, and doesn't rely on laxatives at all.

It is a three-day fasting cleanse. If you have problems fasting completely, the cleanse would also work if you simply do a juice fast or a lemon juice and maple syrup liquid cleanse. On the first two days of the fast you take the following every hour while awake:

- 2 capsules Proactazyme

- 1 capsule High Potency Protease

You can also take the above every 2 hours if taking supplements every hour is too intense for you.

On the third day of the fast, you add probiotics and Colloidal Minerals to start a rebuilding process. You take 2 capsules of Bifidophilus Flora force with the first dose of enzymes. Then, one or two hours later, you take one ounce of colloidal minerals with the next dose of enzymes. You alternative taking probiotics and Colloidal Minerals throughout the day.

On the fourth day, you resume eating. The cleanse is done.

After hearing about this cleanse I've discovered that whenever I feel stuffed, bloated or constipated, all I have to do is stop eating, start drinking lots of liquids and take enzymes every hour and usually within just a few hours, my system is clear. It's a very simple, but effective cleansing technique and works very well for people with spastic colons.

The Once-a-Day Cleanse

Many people have found Ivy's Recipe (see sidebar below) to be an effective daily cleansing program. I've modified her concepts and tried a number of different approaches to this "once-a-day cleanse." Taking a cleansing drink with some cleansing herbs every morning is something I find beneficial as part of a day-to-day health maintenance program.

Ivy's Recipe

Ivy Bridge, an herbalist in Tustin, California has long recommended a once a day cleansing program called Ivy's Recipe. Many people have found this simple cleanse very beneficial. Her program is:

- 2 Tablespoons of. Aloe Vera Juice

- 2 Tablespoons of. Liquid Chlorophyll

- 1 heaping teaspoon of. Psyllium Hulls Combination

These ingredients are blended in a glass of apple juice and taken first thing in the morning. Ivy also recommended taking 2 capsules of cascara sagrada, but I recommend this only if the bowels are not moving at least 2-3 times per day.

The Liquid Cleanse formula could also be taken in place of the cascara sagrada.

Here's a basic "recipe" which you can modify to suit your individual needs.

- 2 Tablespoons of Aloe Vera, Noni and/or Thai-Go

- 2 Tablespoons of Liquid Chlorophyll

- 1 heaping teaspoon of Fiber Blend (Everybody's Fiber, Nature's Three or LOCLO)

These ingredients are blended in a glass of fruit juice and taken first thing in the morning before breakfast. Good juices to use include apple, pear, apricot, peach and pineapple. Orange juice and grapefruit juice usually don't work as well for some reason. Organic juice is preferable. You should also take the following along with the fiber drink:

- 2-4 capsules of a Digestive Enzyme or Enzyme Cleansing Formula (Proactazyme, Bowel Detox, or Small Intestine Detox)

- 2 capsules of a General Cleansing Formula or Hepatic Formula (All Cell Detox, Enviro-Detox, Milk Thistle Combo or Liver Balance)

There are no hard and fast rules here. There are many options available and there is no harm in experimenting with what is best for each individual. The important thing is to assist your body in letting go of the burden of toxins it is carrying around.

Enemas and Colonics

Sometimes one needs to cleanse the colon more quickly. Opening the bowel is the fastest way to relieve most fevers, colds, flu, congestion and acute ailments. It can also rapidly relieve bloated and stuffy feelings, which sometimes happen during a colon cleanse.

The fastest way to open the bowel is with an enema or colonic. These are simple procedures and, properly done, both enemas and colonics are safe and effective. For a colonic, you will need to find a professional colon therapist or purchase a colonic board you can use at home. I've had colonics before, and highly recommend them if they are available in your area.

An enema is something that can be easily done at home. All you need is to purchase an enema bucket or bag. If you have trouble finding one at your local drugstore (I did), you can purchase enema equipment on line at www.enemabag.com or www.enemasupply.com. If you need to give an enema to a baby or a young child, you will want to use a bulb syringe instead of an enema bag.

Enema Solutions

You can use just plain water as an enema solution; however, I recommend that you use purified water, not tap water. An enema is more effective, though, when you use an herbal solution. I've used a wide variety of substances in enemas.

For fevers and infection I've used garlic, made by either blending a clove of fresh garlic in warm water and straining it, or by emptying capsules of garlic powder into warm water and straining it. Other good enema solutions for fevers include teas made of yarrow, catnip, chamomile or peppermint.

A tea made from combination HCP-X is a particularly powerful enema solution. It breaks up "sticky" mucus material and helps expel it rapidly from the colon. It also helps the body pass the rubbery material that forms when toxic bile interacts with the mucilage in fiber. (See Chapter Nine for an explanation of this phenomenon.)

You can also put liquid herbal products into an enema solution. Here are some of the options.

- Blue Vervain (a good choice for fevers, flu, colds and nervousness)

- Catnip and Fennel (good for bloating, gas, indigestion and fevers)

- Echinacea/Goldenseal (good for intestinal infections)

- Lobelia Essence (good for relieving cramping and spastic bowel conditions)

- Oregon Grape (helps detoxify the liver and fight infection)

You can also use a few drops of essential oils in an enema solution, such as lavender oil to relax muscle spasms or tea tree oil for yeast infections and parasites. Always test the enema solution to make sure it is warm, not hot or cold. If you place a couple of drops on your wrist (like testing a baby bottle), it should feel neutral in temperature.

Taking an Enema

Put the enema solution into the enema bucket or bag. Lubricate the tip of the enema syringe thoroughly with a lubricating substance (Golden Salve works well).

When taking an enema lie on your left side first. This allows the solution to move through the rectum and into the descending colon (which is located on the left side of the abdomen). Gently, insert the tip of the enema syringe into the rectum and start the flow of liquid. If you feel any pressure or pain stop the flow. Wait a minute or two to see if the sense of pain or pressure subsides. It may be helpful to massage over the area where you feel pressure or pain.

If the pain or pressure subsides, then resume the flow. If the pain or pressure does not subside, then get up on the toilet and expel the fluid. One doesn't want to "force" the colon to accept more fluid than is comfortable because one doesn't want to stretch the colon. Once you have emptied out, lie down again and repeat the process.

As you are able to get the liquid to move deeper into your colon, you can move from your left side to your back. This allows the liquid to move more freely across the transverse colon (which is located on top of the abdomen just under the ribs). You can also kneel with your head lying on the floor to penetrate this area of the colon.

Finally, you should lie on your right side to allow the fluid to move into your ascending colon (which is located on the right side of your abdomen). Remember that anytime you encounter pressure or pain you should halt the procedure, gently massage the area and wait a minute or so for the sensation of pressure or pain to stop. If it doesn't stop, get up and expel the liquid into the toilet.

If you encounter a spot that you can't seem to get past, you may have an impaction or a spasm in the colon. Massage will help relieve the impaction, and lobelia or lavender oil in the enema solution will relax spasms. You can also apply lobelia or lavender oil topically over the areas where you are experiencing discomfort. You may not be able to clear the entire length of the colon on your first try. It took me quite a few tries before I was able to clear the entire length of the colon.

At the end of the enema, you can put some Acidophilus or Bifidophilus in a small amount of lukewarm water (about 1/2 to 1 cup) and inject it into the rectum. The idea is to not expel this so that it can restore the friendly flora in the intestinal tract. This procedure is known as a rectal injection or retention enema, and can also be used to inject a small amount of white oak bark tea into the rectum for hemorrhoids or rectal bleeding.

Giving a Child an Enema

One can also give an enema to a baby or small child. To do this, place a towel on the floor and lay the child on his or her back or left side on the towel. When doing this with a baby, place a diaper on top of the towel. Explain to the child that this procedure will be uncomfortable, but it will help him or her feel better. Be gentle, but firm. If you were taking the child to the doctor, the child might have to get a shot or have blood drawn which would hurt far more, but you'd probably make them hold still for that anyway. An enema is nowhere near as uncomfortable as a shot, and I've often told children that. I have always talked to my children in a loving, but firm manner when doing this procedure.

Lubricate the anal opening and the tip of the syringe. Fill the syringe with the enema solution by squeezing the syringe and then sucking up the solution. Turn the syringe upright and squeeze any remaining air out of it. Refill the rest of the way, so that the syringe is completely full. Gently insert the tip of the syringe into the anus. Then give a gentle squeeze. If you encounter strong resistance, or the child seems to be in pain, stop squeezing and withdraw the syringe. Make sure you don't "suck" with the syringe as you withdraw.

If nothing comes out, repeat the process again. It may take several tries before anything passes, but don't be concerned, just patient. Putting in a small amount of fluid every five minutes will not hurt the bowel. In fact, small children often get dehydrated when they are feverish from not drinking enough fluids, so the body could be absorbing all of the liquid that you have put into the bowel.

With an older child, tell them they can go "potty" if they feel that they need to. If they don't, then repeat the process. Then wait a minute or two and put a little more fluid in.

With a baby, on the other hand, put a diaper on the baby's bottom after putting one syringe-full into the rectum and then wrap the diaper in a towel. (Enemas can make the stool "runny" and you don't want it to leak onto you.) Then cuddle and hold the baby for a few minutes. Again, if nothing comes out after about ten to twenty minutes, repeat the procedure.

The stool should be soft. If only a small amount of hard stool is passed, you may still need to repeat the process again, until a soft stool passes. The trick is to get the bowel to move freely.

Cleansing the colon can help a wide variety of health problems. It can also improve your complexion, give you more energy, make you feel lighter, and will actually help you lose weight. However, there is more to keeping the colon healthy than just cleansing it, as we'll learn in the next two chapters.

Chapter Seven

The Probiotic Good Guys

Most of us associate bacteria with disease. We think of bacteria as something to be eliminated and destroyed, an attitude that has created an almost obsessive use of disinfectants in our culture. But not all bacteria are bad. It is the action of bacteria, for example, that allows milk to be fermented to create cheese, yogurt and kiefer. Bacteria also create other fermented foods such as sauerkraut, sourdough bread and tofu.

Another benefit of bacteria is that they break down minerals in the soil and make them available to the roots of plants. So, plants need bacteria to be healthy. In fact, one of the reasons plants are often mineral deficient is that modern agricultural methods sterilize the soil with chemicals, killing bacteria which help make minerals available to the roots of a plant.

A plant gets its water nutrients through its roots, which are in the soil. Our "roots," i.e., the place where we absorb water and nutrients, are in the intestinal tract, and bacteria play an important role in our "root" system, too. In fact, there are about three to four pounds of friendly microorganisms living in our intestinal tract, most of them bacteria, which help make certain nutrients available to the body and act as part of our immune system. A proper balance of these microbes is essential to our health.

There is growing evidence that our preoccupation with destroying microbes as a means of preventing disease becomes counterproductive after a point. Overuse of disinfectants in the home increases asthma risk in children, and the constant use of antiseptic soaps has been linked with increased risk for skin infections. Constant use of antibiotics has also been linked with increased susceptibility to infection and reduced immune function. How can this be so?

The reason is that there are bacteria that are good guys, and we live in a symbiotic relationship with these microorganisms. In addition to the internal ecosystem, where billions of microbes are inhabiting our gastrointestinal tract, there is also a surface ecosystem, with billions of additional microbes on the surface of the body. Excessive use of disinfectants destroys the surface ecosystem and increases risk of infection. The same is true for the beneficial bacteria in the intestines. Antibiotics, disinfectants and other germ-killing agents destroy the good guys along with the bad guys, disrupting the balance of the natural ecology and making us more susceptible to a future infection.

The key here is balance. As long as these microbes are in balance, they help us remain healthy. Collectively, the microbes of the internal ecology are known as the intestinal microflora. This internal ecosystem is composed of 400-500 different strains of bacteria and other microorganisms. When it is balanced, it protects against infection and promotes health. When it is imbalanced, it creates the conditions that promote disease.

There are many different species of beneficial bacteria inhabiting our intestines. Many belong to the genus *Lactobacillus*. These include *L. acidophilus*, one of the first strains sold as a supplement. Another genus containing species of friendly bacteria is Bifidobacterium, sometimes referred to as *Bifidophilus*. A third major group belong to the *Streptoccus* genus. There are many others.

The friendly bacteria inhabiting the intestines are called friendly flora or probiotics. "Biotic" is from a Greek word that refers to life. So pro-biotic means "favorable to life". This is in contrast with the word anti-biotic, which literally means "against life".

As has already been established, antibiotics weaken the immune system because they destroy the friendly flora. They may be useful, and necessary, in certain serious infections, but they are routinely over-prescribed for viral conditions on which they have no effect. They are also used in animal feed. Indiscriminately using something that is "against life" is not going to be good for our health, especially when it kills friendly flora that are actually part of the immune system.

Friendly bacteria enhance the immune system in several ways. First of all, they form a sort of living "blanket" that coats the intestinal tract and inhibits other species of microorganisms from "gaining a foothold" on the intestinal mucosa. They compete with other microbes for food, which also holds down the growth of infectious organisms.

Friendly bacteria even produce chemicals that are deadly to harmful forms of bacteria, so they act as natural antibiotic agents against harmful bacteria. Another benefit of friendly bacteria is that they have a stimulating effect on the body's immune system. For instance, animal studies showed that *S. thermophilus* and *L. bulgaricus* increased proliferation of lymphocytes, stimulated B lymphocytes and activated macrophages.

The final and best-known benefit of friendly flora is their ability to prevent yeast such as *Candida albicans* from multiplying out of control. This is one of the primary problems with antibiotics. Antibiotics not only kill harmful bacteria, they also kill the friendly bacteria and encourage yeast overgrowth. Yeasts secrete a toxin that weakens the intestinal membranes and reduces the immune response. Probiotics are the antidote to this side effect of antibiotics, helping to restore a healthy intestinal microflora.

Other Benefits

Protection against infections and enhanced immunity, however, isn't the only benefit the intestinal microflora provide. A number of studies have shown that probiotics can help prevent diarrhea. By taking probiotics with meals when traveling abroad, many people have been able to prevent diarrhea caused by unfamiliar microbes in the food and water.

Probiotics also help overall colon health. They reduce the risk of inflammatory bowel disorders such as colitis, Crohn's disease and irritable bowel syndrome. They also reduce the risk of colon cancer. They should be used as part of a natural therapy plan for these diseases.

Healthy intestinal microflora improve the body's ability to digest fats and proteins. Probiotics synthesize certain vitamins the body needs, including B1, B2, B6, B12, folic acid and biotin. The synthesis of B12 by probiotics is particularly important for vegetarians who are not getting this vitamin in their diets.

The friendly flora also help detoxify certain poisons in the digestive tract. For instance, they help break down ammonia, cholesterol, and excess hormones.

The anthraquinone glycosides in stimulant laxative herbs like cascara sagrada and senna are activated by the intestinal microflora. In fact, these herbs are much less effective if the intestinal microflora is out of balance. Even when used by themselves, probiotics improve colon elimination, helping arrest diarrhea or overcome constipation.

Finally, about 70% of the energy requirements of the intestinal mucosa come from fatty acids produced as a by-product of bacterial fermentation. This means that the intestinal microflora actually helps feed the intestinal lining. This demonstrates how vital this synergistic relationship is to health.

In fact, a healthy intestinal microflora is such an important part of total health, that some health researchers feel it should be considered as an independent body system. The intestinal microflora is a highly adaptable system, as it changes constantly, adapting itself to one's diet and environment. It is easy to see why a balanced intestinal microflora is such an important factor in a healthy body.

Who Needs Probiotics?

Most people living in western society can benefit from taking probiotics. Since antibiotics are the worst culprit for throwing intestinal flora out of balance, anyone who has had an antibiotic should take a probiotic supplement. Don't forget that antibiotics are also hidden in meat and dairy foods. So, if you use animal products, periodic supplementation with probiotics is very important.

Chlorine and other antibacterial chemicals added to drinking water also upset the balance of the microflora. Pesticides and herbicides present in our foods also have disruptive effects.

People who suffer from yeast infections of any kind, including athlete's foot, jock itch, vaginal yeast infections and nail fungus needs to restore balance to their intestinal microflora using probiotics.

People with weak immune systems, frequent respiratory infections and congestion, food or respiratory allergies, inflammatory bowel disorders, skin eruptions, constipation or intestinal infections may also see health improvements when taking probiotics.

People who travel can avoid infections from foreign food and water by taking probiotics with meals. Probiotics can also be given to children and infants to reduce the risk of infection. In short, probiotics are a basic health-building supplement, as important for most Americans as a multivitamin.

A variety of probiotics are available for different needs and purposes. One can improve one's intestinal flora by eating plain yogurt (preferably organic) with live bacterial cultures and other fermented foods with live cultures (such as fresh sauerkraut or kim chi). One can also take probiotic supplements. Here are four probiotic supplements you can use and the potential benefits of each.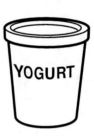

Acidophilus

Acidophilus contains the species Lactobacillus acidophilus in a dairy-free base. *L. acidophilus* is one of the major bacteria in the intestinal microflora of both the small and large intestines. These bacteria are also present in the mouth and vagina. Some of the benefits of acidophilus include:

• Enhancing the digestion of milk sugar (lactose) by producing lactase. This helps prevent lactose intolerance of dairy foods.

• Aiding in the digestion of other nutrients.

• Creating lactic acid and other inhibitory substances that suppress undesirable strains of microbes in the intestines.

• Producing natural antibacterial substances that inhibit hostile bacteria.

• Helping to break down and eliminate cholesterol.

• Reducing proliferation of yeasts such as *Candida albicans*.

Acidophilus is probably the most widely used probiotic supplement, but with so many other species available, it is often better to use a supplement that contains several strains.

Bifidophilus Flora Force

The Bifidophilus Flora Force supplement also contains *L. acidophilus*, but includes three other species of friendly bacteria—*L. caseii, L. rhamnosus,* and *Bifidobacterium longum.* This product is in a base of fructo-oligosaccharides, which serve as food for the bacteria and aid their implantation in the colon. This supplement provides the benefits of acidophilus with added benefits of the other strains.

B. longum is a very abundant organism found in the large intestine. It plays an important role in crowding out pathological organisms and yeast. In clinical studies, it has been found to reduce the frequency of gastrointestinal disorders such as diarrhea and nausea during antibiotic use. B. longum also helps balance pH levels in the intestines, further inhibiting undesirable bacterial growth. The bifido strains of bacteria also appear to suppress excess cholesterol production and help produce certain B vitamins.

L. casei is a transient bacteria found in the large intestine and mouth. It is found in milk and cheese. It has effects similar to L. acidophilus. *L. rhamnosus* is found primarily in the small intestine and the vagina, where it helps inhibit bacterial infections. It is a species with a prolific growth pattern and has a high tolerance to bile salts (one of the digestive secretions that destroys bacteria). Research suggests it may be helpful in reducing gut sensitivity and helping with eczema and food allergies.

L-Reuteri

Lactobacillus reuteri is a strain of lactobacillus that is stable enough to allow it to be placed in a chewable tablet that does not require refrigeration. This strain of bacteria is found in breast milk and is indigenous to the human digestive tract. It is much more viable than *L. acidophilus* or *B. longum* in surviving stomach acid and bile salts, so it is more effective than other probiotics when taken orally. It also adheres better to the intestinal lining.

With over 50 years of clinical research involving over 1000 scientific articles, *L. reuteri* is clinically proven to provide a variety of health benefits. *L. reuteri* is unique among probiotic bacteria in its ability to form an antimicrobial substance called reuterin. This substance can inhibit and/or prevent the growth of many different types of microorganisms, both gram-positive and gram-negative bacteria, fungi and protozoa. It may also play a role in neutralizing toxins, including carcinogens.

A more recent discovery is a substance it produces called reutericyclin, which also combats other bacteria. So, it supports the growth of other friendly bacteria, while inhibiting other unfriendly organisms. Thus, it promotes a healthier balance of microflora in the intestines.

L. reuteri increases surface area in the microvilli of the intestinal tract. This improves mineral and nutrient absorption. It also helps break down cholesterol. *L. reuteri* is clinically proven to enhance colon health in children, reducing bowel distress, irregularity and infections. It also helps reduce allergic reactions in children.

Because of its unique properties, L-Reuteri is one of the best probiotic supplements to take after a round of antibiotics to restore balance to the intestinal flora.

Probiotic Eleven

You've probably heard of broad-spectrum antibiotics, a term that refers to an antibiotic that kills a broad range of bacteria. Well, Probiotic Eleven is a broad spectrum probiotic, because it contains eleven different species of friendly bacteria. In addition to the *L. acidophilus, B. longum, L. rhamnosus,* and *L. casei* we've already discussed, Probiotic Eleven also contains the following.

B. bifidus is a probiotic organism residing primarily in the mucus membrane lining of the colon and vaginal tract. It prevents invading pathogenic bacteria from attaching to the intestinal wall. It also enhances mineral assimilation.

L. brevis is a bacteria found in milk, kefir, cheese, and sauerkraut. It helps produce lactic acid and natural antibacterial agents that inhibit unfriendly strains of microorganisms. It also helps with the synthesis of vitamins D and K.

L. bulgaricus is a transient, but important, bacteria in the ecology of the intestines. It is used along with *Streptococcus thermophilus* to create yogurt and is found in both yogurt and cheese. It helps digest lactase (milk sugar) to improve tolerance to dairy products. It also produces lactic acid to inhibit the growth of harmful microbes.

L. plantarum is another transient bacteria found in dairy products, sauerkraut and pickled vegetables. They are another lactic acid producing strain of bacteria. *S. thermophilus* is the other bacteria in yogurt culture. It also produces lactase to digest milk sugar. In fact, it is the best strain for helping break down dairy products.

B. infantis is an important strain that helps stimulate the immune system. It has been observed to have action against pathological organisms like clostridia, salmonella and shigella. *L. salivarius* helps normalize the intestinal microflora and may inhibit *H. pylori*, the bacteria associated with stomach ulcers.

Using Probiotics

Always take probiotics after any round of antibiotics or after doing any cleanse. Probiotics should also be taken as part of a health-building program for anyone who is chronically ill or who has weak immunity.

Generally speaking, the best times to take probiotics are first thing in the morning or on an empty stomach right before going to bed. Follow directions on the bottle.

Probiotics can also be injected directly into the rectum by mixing them with a little tepid (not hot) water and injecting it directly into the rectum. They can be sprinkled into a diaper to help rashes in small children and may be applied topically for yeast infections on the skin.

Finally, these friendly bacteria won't "stick around" in a colon where the environment is toxic or where there are too many parasites which have taken hold of the body. So, it may be necessary to do some colon cleansing (see previous chapters) or some parasite cleansing (see next chapter) in order to reestablish a healthy intestinal flora.

Chapter Eight

The Parasitic Bad Guys

As we've just learned, even when we're healthy, our intestinal tract is a zoo of living creatures. Hopefully, we're playing host to friendly organisms, but sometimes the creatures in our intestinal zoo are dangerous critters to our health. Parasites are far more common than people realize. They can be picked up from household pets, foreign travel, contaminated water or food, or open wounds.

Parasite problems are so evasive to regular medical investigation that no one can accurately estimate how much of the population may be afflicted by parasites. Present estimates range from 25-80% for Americans.

Parasites aren't just worms, either. Harmful microbes including giardia, candida and amoebas can also be classified as parasites. When organisms like these are included, it is likely that at least two-thirds of all Americans have at least one type of parasite in their body.

Symptoms usually depend on the type of parasite, but generally they include nervousness, grinding teeth at night (especially children), constant hunger with unsatisfied appetite, itching rectum, severe health problems that develop after foreign travel, and constant gastrointestinal problems like nausea, diarrhea and sensitive bowels. Parasites can also cause chronic fatigue, bad breath, anemia, ulcers, itching, chronic nose picking, mood swings and insomnia.

Parasites can be very hard to diagnose. A stool analysis may or may not reveal the existence of parasites because, even if parasites are present in the bowel, they may or may not be present in any particular stool sample. Parasites may also be in other body tissues and not show up in the bowel.

Even when diagnosed correctly, parasites can be very hard to eliminate. It takes very powerful medications to kill parasites and typically, those medications are toxic to healthy tissue as well. Even some of the stronger antiparasitic herbs have some toxicity. However, our approach to parasites is going to be only partially effective if we focus only on trying to kill them.

While parasites may be present in many chronic diseases, they aren't really the root cause. All parasites require a supportive host environment in order to survive. If the host environment isn't conducive to its growth, a parasite will have a difficult time gaining a foothold.

So, we also need to change the host environment to make it unfriendly for the growth of parasites. This is where herbs can excel over chemical drugs. While they may not be as strong at directly killing the parasites, they are exceptionally good at helping to alter the host environment and making it unfriendly to parasites. When combined with general cleansing, improved diet, and other healthy habits, herbal parasite cleanses can be very effective.

Know the Enemy

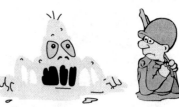

One of the most common parasitical organisms in North Americans is *Candida albicans*, a species of yeast. Candida is present even in healthy colons, but it multiplies out of control when the acidophilus and bifidophilus in the intestinal tract are killed by antibiotics. Yeast overgrowth causes immune weakness, cravings for sugar, frequent colds, sore throats, sinus infections and fatigue. It may become systemic, resulting in finger and toenail infections, vaginal yeast infections and itching skin. Ringworm is actually a fungal infection of the skin and can often be treated topically.

Another common single-celled parasite is giardia. Giardia is picked up by drinking contaminated water and causes diarrhea. Amoebas are another intestinal parasite that cause severe diarrhea (amoebic dysentery). Although not commonly thought of as a parasite, H. pylori is a bacteria that can infect the stomach and intestines and is associated with ulcers.

There are also several types of worms that may infect the body. Tapeworms are probably the biggest, and can range from one inch to thirty feet (yes, feet) long. They are believed to live up to 25 years and can cause weight loss, abdominal pain, vomiting and diarrhea.

Roundworms (including protozoa and flukes), ascarids, and hookworms are contagious intestinal parasites. They are shaped like earthworms but smaller. Hookworms can also infect the feet and cause itching there. The smaller roundworms can infect muscles and also damage the heart and nervous system. Large roundworms and whipworms can cause respiratory problems and may crawl up into the throat and, in extreme cases, exit through the mouth or nose.

Pinworms show up as short white threads less than half an inch long. Pinworms can cause severe anal itching and trouble sleeping. They may leave through the rectum at night to lay eggs. They are the most common worm problem for young children and are easily passed around the family.

Precautions to prevent spreading worms would include washing bed linens, bed clothes and underwear of entire family, having infected child take daily morning showers to remove eggs deposited in the perianal region during the night, using disinfectants daily on the toilet seat and bathtub, and being sure everybody washes their hands (and fingernails of those infected) before meals. In fact, the entire family should do a parasite cleanse.

These are not the only parasites it is possible to have. There are about 1,000 known types of parasites. Fortunately, natural remedies are fairly broad acting, so it isn't necessary to know exactly what parasites are present in order to get rid of them.

Choose Your Weapons

Herbs that work against parasites are classified as anthelmintics/vermifuges (expel or destroy worms) or parasiticides (kill parasites). Some herbs are directly toxic to parasites. Some "stun" or relax them so that they can't stay in place and are eliminated with regular bowel movements. Other herbs clean up the host terrain, making the environment unfriendly to parasites, encouraging them to leave. Effective herbal therapy for parasites involves a combination of all of these strategies.

There are many herbs which can help fight parasites. For instance, Garlic, especially if taken raw (so that it still has plenty of the stinky allicin), is useful against bacteria, yeast and worms. High Potency Garlic uses a chlorophyll coating to reduce odor and prevent the tablet from breaking down until it reaches the small intestine. Each tablet has a total allicin potential of 1,200 mg. This is about the same as about four cloves of fresh garlic.

Black walnut is another reliable herb for parasites. Tourists in tropical climates should take black walnut frequently to avoid diarrhea due to unclean water. Black walnut is an effective astringent and helps tighten tissues and restore tone to bowel tissues. Black Walnut Extract (liquid) is especially easy for children to take.

Plants in the Artemisia genus include some of the strongest antiparasitic herbs available. These include wormwood and mugwort. Wormwood is very bitter and aromtic. It contains thujone, an oil that can stun roundworms. Both wormwood and mugwort are slightly toxic, and should be avoided by small children and pregnant or nursing mothers. They have bowel cleansing and powerful anthelmintic effects and are safest when used as part of a formula (such as Artemesia Combination).

Olive Leaf Extract is widely used against fungal infections, the malaria parasite, and other parasitic infections. As a "good side effect," olive leaf extract can dramatically improve immune system function and is used to fight viruses and prevent bacterial infections.

Other single herbal remedies for parasites include goldenseal, which is an excellent remedy for giardia, and Activated Charcoal, which is helpful for severe diarrhea associated with parasites. Pau d'arco, olive leaf, garlic and oregano are all good single remedies for yeast infections.

Antiparastic herbs work best when taken in combination with herbs that help to cleanse the bowels and tissues. Para-Cleanse is a convenient, pre-packaged parasite cleansing program, which contains all of the previously mentioned herbs and more. (See sidebar for more information.)

Doing a Parasite Cleanse

Some parasites reproduce through a multi-stage life cycle. Eggs may be protected in a durable shell, so that even if you take an antiparasitic product now, those eggs will survive and hatch, and the larvae will promptly create a reinfestation. The solution is to use a program that repeats the treatment several times. Since family members often share

---

ParaCleanse: An Effective Parasite Cleansing Program

ParaCleanse contains the following herbal products: Herbal Pumpkin, Yeast/Fungal Detox, Artemesia Combination, and Paw Paw Cell Reg.

Herbal Pumpkin is a reliable formula that has been used successfully for many years against a wide variety of parasites. It contains the antiparasitic herbs pumpkin seeds and black walnut combined with liver and gastrointestinal cleansing herbs like cascara sagrada, violet leaves, marshmallow and slippery elm bark

Yeast/Fungal Detox contains several anti-fungal herbs and nutrients, including: caprylic acid, sodium propionate, sorbic acid, oregano, garlic and pau d'arco. These are combined with immune-enhancing selenium, zinc and Echinacea purpurea.

Artemisia Combination contains two species of Artemisia: mugwort and wormwood, powerful antiparasitics mentioned earlier. It also contains elecampane, clove, garlic, ginger, spearmint, turmeric and olive leaf, which help fight yeast, parasites, bacterial infections and improve gastro-intestinal function and tone.

Finally, Paw Paw Cell-Reg adds the special property of killing parasites by reducing their ability to create life energy. Although Paw Paw Cell-Reg is primarily used to fight abnormal cell growth, it is also effective against parasites. It works by reducing the ability of the mitochondria ("energy factories") in cells to convert nutrients into energy for their own life functions. Specifically, it blocks the production of adenosine triphosphate (ATP), a cellular energy storage molecule that causes single-celled organisms and worms to die.

---

parasites with each other, best results are obtained when all family members follow the program at the same time.

Start by doing a regular colon cleanse as described in chapter six. The Tiao He Cleanse or CleanStart would be good choices. This removes old fecal material that may be present and gets the colon in a healthier condition, which makes it easier to get rid of the parasites.

Next, do one 10-day Para-Cleanse Program. This involves taking one packet of the Para-Cleanse 15 minutes before breakfast and another 15 minutes before dinner for ten days. Be sure to drink plenty of water. If your bowels don't move regularly, you may wish to add some fiber or a stimulant laxative like LBS II or cascara sagrada.

After completing the first round of the parasite cleanse wait one week. It might be a good idea to do a regular colon cleanse during this week. The one-week break allows any eggs that may have been present to hatch. So, now do a second 10-day round of the Para-Cleanse program.

For really serious parasite problems, this process can be repeated two or three times, following the Para-Cleanse Program for 10 days, then taking a one-week break.

At the end of the program, be sure to take probiotics like Acidophilus or Bifidophilus Flora Force after the strong herbs of an antiparasitic just as you would after using antibiotics. This assures that healthful bacteria, which may also have been killed, are replanted. These will help to displace parasites and prevent reinfestation by other organisms.

Special Parasite Cleanses

In addition to the Para-Cleanse program, you can also use the following "do-it-yourself" parasite cleanse.

Worm Cleanse

This cleanse is aimed more specifically at worms.

- 2 capsules Herbal Pumpkin three times per day
- 2 capsules Black Walnut three times per day

- 2 capsules Artemisia Combination three times per day

- 1 High Potency Garlic twice daily

- 2 capsules Hi-Potency Protease three times daily

This program should be repeated for 14 days (2 weeks), then followed by a one-week break. After the one-week break a second 14-day round of antiparasitics should be taken. This could be repeated a third time, if necessary.

Yeast/Fungal Cleanse

For yeast infections, a sample "do-it-yourself" cleansing program would be:

- 1 Capryllic Acid Combo or 1 Yeast/Fungal Detox twice daily

- 2 Pau D'Arco three times daily

- 1 High Potency Garlic twice daily

- 2 capsules of a general cleansing formula (such as Enviro-Detox or All Cell Detox) three times daily

- A fiber drink in the morning before breakfast using Everybody's Fiber.

A yeast or candida cleanse should be done for at least two to three weeks, and perhaps as long as a month. During the cleanse the person should avoid all simple sugars and refined grains (white flour, white rice, etc.). Even whole grains and starchy foods like potatoes should be minimized as yeasts like to feed on simple sugars and starch. The diet should consist primarily of fresh fruits, vegetables and lean meats.

Giardia

America has prided herself on excellent municipal water systems and inspection standards. However, besides chemical pollution, the parasite *Giardia lamblia* seems to be taking the world by storm, doubling every five years. Drinking water from open streams is a common way to be infected by Giardia cysts, but food and hand-to-mouth contact may also transmit the disease.

Ten grams of goldenseal daily for ten days has been proven effective in ridding the body of Giardia. The addition of ginger (1 three times daily) and activated charcoal (2 two or three times daily) can help eliminate the diarrhea that accompanies this infection.

Bacteria

Gastro Health can help with *H. pylori* and other bacterial infections in the intestinal tract. It contains a proprietary blend of herbs that have been proven effective against these bacteria including cloves, licorice, and elecampane. These herbs also serve to soothe inflammation and feed friendly bacteria in the intestines.

Additional Steps

It isn't enough to just try to kill the parasites. One has to restore a healthy environment to the gastrointestinal tract. So, after any parasite cleanse it's important to take digestive enzymes such as Proactazyme Plus or High Potency Protease with meals in order to help food digest better. Small Intestine Detox can also be used to remove mucus from the intestines.

One also has to replace the good guys, the friendly probiotics, that are supposed to dominate the intestinal tract. Good supplements for this are Acidophilus and Bifidophilus Flora Force. L. Reuteri is particularly helpful in getting rid of yeast.

Parasites like yeast, bacteria, etc. cause intestinal inflammation which causes the intestinal membranes to lose tone and "leak" toxins into the blood and lymph. Following a parasite cleanse it is important to restore tone to the intestinal tract. Some of the herbs that will help to reduce leaky gut include licorice, una d'gato or cat's claw, chamomile, kudzu, slippery elm and plantain. Two great formulas for this are Intestinal Soothe and Build and Kudzu/St. John's wort.

Chapter Nine

Liver and Gallbladder Cleansing

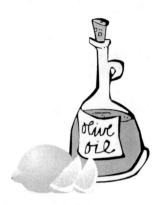

Up until now, we've concentrated on learning how to "sweep" the body's main chimney, the colon and gastrointestinal tract, clear of debris. While the cleanses we've discussed have also contained substances which help to detoxify through the liver, kidneys, lymphatics and so forth, we're now ready to learn how to do specialized cleanses. Sometimes, we need to focus special effort on strengthening specific organs of detoxification, such as the liver, which is the subject of this chapter.

As we've already discussed, the liver is the most important organ of internal detoxification and works hand in hand with the colon. When the colon and intestines are toxic, that is, filled with waste material that is not being eliminated quickly enough from the body, some of this toxic material is absorbed into the blood stream. All the blood from the intestinal tract is transported first to the liver, which acts as our second line of defense against toxins.

The liver is an amazing organ. It performs over 500 functions and contains hundreds of enzyme systems that can process foodstuffs or break toxins down into simpler compounds that the body can eliminate. The liver is doing its best to handle the pesticide residues, food additives, drugs and other chemicals it is being bombarded with in modern society, and it's doing this for many people while being fed a diet of "junk food" lacking in the critical nutrients it needs. No wonder so many people's livers need cleansing and rebuilding.

One of the methods the liver can utilize when dealing with a toxin is to flush it back into the digestive tract via the gallbladder. This "toxic bile" irritates the upper part of the small intestines, creating nausea, vomiting and diarrhea. This procedure can be thought of as a kind of self-cleansing "chimney fire" in the digestive tract. It is called a "liver crisis" by some natural healers. The nausea, vomiting, diarrhea and aching feeling that accompany this liver crisis or 24-hour flu are the result of the efforts of the liver to detoxify the body. Morning sickness is another form of liver crisis that occurs in pregnant women as their bodies try to flush toxins to protect the developing baby.

Mucilaginous herbs, fiber or small amounts of activated charcoal, can absorb the toxic bile being released from the liver and keep it from recycling (i.e., being reabsorbed into the intestines and transported back to the liver). This is an important part of what is happening on a cleanse (see "Bile and Fiber" below), and is one of the many reasons fiber supplements are so beneficial.

Bile and Fiber

Many people who are taking fiber products on a cleanse will notice that they pass a rubbery sort of material that is thick and ropy. Many believe this is material that was adhered to (or encrusted on) the lining of the colon. However, this isn't the case. Modern diagnostic techniques allow doctors to look directly into the colon using fiber optics, and even natural healers who have been able to participate in this procedure have assured me that there is no encrusted lining on the colon. (Quite honestly, such a lining would kill you in a few days by inhibiting absorption of water and nutrients.)

Also, this material does not pass simply by taking laxatives. It only passes when one is taking fiber, and herein lies the secret to what this material is. The rubbery material that passes from some people during a cleanse is formed when toxic bile interacts with the mucilage in herbs like psyllium and marshmallow. The fiber absorbs the toxic bile and it turns into this rubber material. I learned this fact from Mark Pederson, a talented chemist and author of *Nutritional Herbology*.

This is why fiber is so important. Without fiber, this toxic material being released from the liver could be absorbed back into the blood stream and carried back to the liver to be recycled. Fiber ensures that the material is flushed out of the body—for good!

Herbs can also be used that strengthen the liver and promote more bile flow to flush the liver more quickly. These herbs are called chologagogues, and include artichoke leaf, blessed thistle, turmeric, dandelion, barberry, fringetree and milk thistle. When used in combination with dietary fiber, cholagogues will help to remove fat-soluble toxins from the body, while helping to lower cholesterol and triglycerides. This is because the primary use for cholesterol in the body is to manufacture bile to help break down fats.

When fiber is lacking in the diet, cholesterol released from the gallbladder can be reabsorbed and transported back to the liver. As it recycles through the gallbladder it concentrates and forms gallstones. When this happens, a gall bladder flush may be in order. In fact, doing a colon cleanse along with a gall bladder flush is one of the fastest ways to reduce high cholesterol levels.

Directions for a Gall Bladder Flush

Here's how a gallbladder flush is done. Start by fasting for 24 to 48 hours on fresh, raw apple juice or fresh squeezed grapefruit juice to clear the colon. Malic acid, an ingredient in the apple juice, helps soften the stones, but persons with hypoglycemia or yeast infections will do better on grapefruit juice. If using grapefruit, juice take Fibralgia, which contains malic acid and magnesium, for a similar stone softening effect.

Just before going to bed at the close of the fast, mix 1/2 cup of olive oil and 1/2 cup of lemon (or grapefruit) juice and drink the mixture. Mix the olive oil and juice together thoroughly, just like you would shake up a salad dressing. The lemon juice cuts the olive oil and makes it more palatable. It's not as bad as one might think. If you can get past the smell, the taste is all right.

After drinking this mixture, lie on your right side for a half hour before going to sleep. In the morning, if you don't have a bowel movement, take an enema. This procedure may need to be repeated two or three days in a row.

Generally, you will pass some dark black or green objects that look like shriveled peas the day after drinking the olive oil and lemon juice. Some people think these objects are the gallstones, but they are not.

Gallstones that can be passed are much smaller than this, generally less than 2 millimeters in diameter. About five different herbalists and naturopaths have told me that they have taken these objects to the lab for chemical analysis and it turns out they are composed of soap.

So, just like the rubber material on a colon cleanse is formed by the interaction of toxic bile with mucilaginous fiber, these dark black or green objects are created by the interaction of toxic bile and the olive oil. The large amount of oil being taken at once causes large amounts of bile to be flushed through the gallbladder in an attempt to digest the fats. This lowers cholesterol (because cholesterol is a major component of bile), and causes smaller stones to be expelled. Some of the materials used in the gallbladder flush can also help dissolve bigger gallstones when used regularly in smaller quantities. In fact, just taking fiber and some of the stronger cholagogue herbs regularly will help to dissolve and expel gallstones.

I've done the gallbladder flush myself several times and used it with numerous clients. There are a number of versions of this procedure, but they all rely on olive oil, which appears to help dissolve stones even when taken in smaller doses over a more extended period of time. One natural healer I met used six tablespoons of olive oil and 6 tablespoons of lemon juice every night for 30 days to flush the gallbladder. He claimed this was gentler, but worked just as well.

Another variation, one I learned from a midwife friend of mine, is to take a dose of Epsom salt about two or three hours prior to taking the olive oil and lemon juice. Follow the directions on the box of Epsom salts as per the dosage. Epsom salt acts as a natural laxative and the magnesium is helpful for dissolving any stones that may contain calcium.

One can also take cholagogue herbs during the fast to increase the flow of bile and improve the effectiveness of the procedure. Herbs to consider include dandelion root, barberry bark, yellow dock root, turmeric and fringetree bark. Any of these can be taken before attempting the gallbladder flush to increase its effectiveness, or afterwards to continue improving gallbladder function. Gall Bladder Formula is a mild cholagogue and antispasmodic and can be taken during the juice fast, or for several months to help flush the liver and gallbladder. Take 2 capsules 3 times daily.

There is a small chance that a very large stone could become lodged in the bile ducts, which would require that surgery be performed to remove the gallbladder. However, thousands of people have used this procedure and I have only had one case reported to me where this happened. Since this procedure is typically done as an alternative to surgery, I believe it is well worth trying, as a person can go ahead with the surgery if the procedure fails to relieve the problem.

The Liver and Fat Soluble Toxins

One of the reasons the liver and gallbladder are so important to address in cleansing is because many toxins are not water-soluble. This includes mercury, formaldehyde and many petrochemicals, such as gasoline. These chemicals can only be dissolved in fats. Many household cleaning products, cosmetics, dry cleaning solvents, and agricultural chemicals fall into this category. So, when these chemicals get into the body, the body has to attach them to fats in order to transport and eliminate them.

This is one of the primary reasons why people's cholesterol rises. The body is increasing cholesterol production in order to mop up environmental toxins and protect sensitive tissues like the nerves. This also explains why lower cholesterol levels are associated with an increased risk of cancer.

If the eliminative channels can't get rid of these fat soluble toxins, then they going to get stored—in fat. When you break down the fat, then the chemicals are going to be released into the blood stream, causing lots of problems if the liver and eliminative organs aren't strong enough to handle them. This is why cleansing is so important to weight loss.

This is also why essential fatty acid supplements are often needed to help with detoxification. Flax seed oil, Super GLA or Super Omega-3 EPA are good choices. Hi-Lipase can help the body digest and process these healthy fats, while SF and chickweed relieve fatty congestion in the liver and help the liver deal with fat-soluble toxins.

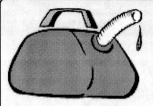

Toxic Reaction to Gasoline

I had a personal experience with how the body handles these fat-soluble toxins one summer while I was camping with my kids. We arrived at our campsite after dark. I was wearing shorts and in my attempt to fill the Coleman lantern with white gas, I spilled gasoline all over my legs. I knew this wasn't good, but I wiped it off and didn't think too much about it, trusting my body was healthy enough to deal with it.

On the second night of our camping trip, I woke up in the middle of the night with my head swimming and my stomach churning. I thought I had food poisoning. After several hours of dozing in and out of sleep, and trying to drink some water to flush my system, I finally managed to throw up. What I threw up was mostly bile.

None of my kids were sick, so I realized that I couldn't have had food poisoning. What was the problem then? I finally realized that it was the white gas. My body had been healthy enough to deal with it. It had used cholesterol in my bloodstream to grab hold of the chemical and transport it to my liver, where it was emptied into the bile ducts (that's how the body eliminates cholesterol). This made me nauseous and caused me to throw up, eliminating the chemical from my system.

If just one exposure to a fat-soluble chemical like gasoline could do that, think about what repeated exposure to solvents, cleaning solutions, beauty parlor chemicals, paints, mercury, and a host of other fat soluble chemicals over a long period of time can do. One can see why keeping the liver healthy is so important in today's chemical-laden world.

Protecting the Liver from Toxins

Keeping one's liver in good working condition can be a challenge in our modern world. The liver must process many of the chemicals we encounter in our environment, from pesticide residues and food additives to chemicals in the air we breath and the water we drink. The diet of highly refined and nutrient-depleted foods that most Americans eat challenges the liver to keep up with its load. Add to that the consumption of hepatotoxic (liver poisoning) substances like alcohol and many drugs, which can do serious damage to the liver.

Moderate liver dysfunction is involved in a wide variety of health problems including digestive upset, nausea, diarrhea, poor fat digestion, headaches, hot flashes, hypoglycemia, PMS symptoms, uterine fibroids, prostate problems, skin eruptions like acne and hives, allergies, anemia and high cholesterol levels. Liver stress is probably a part of many chronic diseases including cardiovascular disease, diabetes, arthritis and even cancer.

Fortunately, herbs can do a lot to help prevent damage to the liver from these environmental toxins. One herb in particular has been well researched in this regard, and that is milk thistle. Studies have shown that milk thistle has a protective effect on liver tissue, even in cases of chemical poisoning. It keeps toxins absorbed by the intestines from damaging the liver while it works to neutralize them.

Protecting the Liver with Milk Thistle Combination

Milk Thistle Combination contains nutrients, known to aid liver function and help the liver resist environmental toxins. These include a standardized extract of milk thistle, which contains 80% silymarin, an antioxidant complex that strengthens the integrity of liver tissue and protects it against a wide variety of hepatotoxic substances.

Dandelion also supports liver function by increasing bile production and enhancing liver detoxification. N-Acetyl-Cysteine, a substance built on the amino acid cysteine, helps the liver make glutathione, a powerful antioxidant that increases cellular detoxification. This helps the liver by preventing free radical damage and enhancing its ability to remove waste products and irritants.

This formula also contains several vitamins that are needed for the liver's detoxification processes. Beta carotene and vitamin C are needed in large amounts by the liver. Choline bitartrate and inositol are lipotropic; they increase the transportation and metabolism of fat in the liver. This reduces fatty liver congestion, which is common in developed countries. These are "unofficial" B vitamins that protect against liver scarring and help prevent cirrhosis and high cholesterol.

Milk Thistle Combination is a great blend to protect the liver from chemicals in the environment, and a good daily supplement for anyone whose job requires them to work around chemicals on a regular basis.

In Europe, milk thistle is used as an antidote to poisoning by death cap mushrooms (Amanita sp.). These mushrooms contain powerful hepatotoxins that damage liver tissue when they are absorbed into the blood stream. Of course, the liver tries to flush them out through the bile (causing nausea, vomiting and diarrhea), but the toxins are easily reabsorbed. On each pass through the liver they damage more tissue, killing the patient. Milk thistle inhibits the liver damage, thus helping the body flush the mushroom toxin with less tissue damage. It is helpful for other toxins, too. In fact, I think anyone who works around fat-soluble chemicals of any kind (painters, hair stylists, dry cleaners, auto mechanics, etc.) ought to take essential fatty acids (such as flax seed oil or Super GLA oil) and Milk Thistle Combination every day to protect their liver. Milk thistle can also help swimmers who swim in chlorinated water to have more energy. (See sidebar on Milk Thistle Combination.)

There are other supplements that can also assist the liver in being more efficient at detoxification. These include the general cleansing formulas we've already discussed, All Cell Detox and Enviro-Detox, and some specific liver formulas, including Liver Balance, Blood Build and Liver Cleanse Formula. Nutrients like alpha-lipoic acid, n-aceytl-cysteine and Sam-e will also help with liver detoxification.

Blood Purifiers and Skin Conditions

There is also a strong connection between the liver and the skin. The oil ducts in the skin can also be used to eliminate fat-soluble toxins. So, skin problems such as acne, pimples, pox, dry skin, eczema, dermatitis, and itching may indicate the liver is overburdened with toxic fat and can't handle the load. So, the skin is now acting as a safety valve, an overflow for the excess toxicity. Traditional herbalists saw these problems as signs of impure blood and used remedies called blood purifiers to promote healing. Most herbs classified as blood purifiers work on the liver, with secondary benefits to the lymphatics and/or urinary system.

As we've discussed, toxins from the intestinal tract are absorbed into the bloodstream and transported through the liver. The liver will try to neutralize these toxic substances or flush them back into the intestinal tract via the gallbladder. However, if the liver can't handle the toxic load, then the toxins get into the general circulation. So, the blood becomes "impure."

At this point, the endocrine system kicks into gear to stimulate elimination of these toxins through other channels. Depending on the relative strength of various glands and the type of toxin involved, the body may choose to push these toxins out of the body through the skin, the kidneys, the mucus membranes of the respiratory tract, or, in the case of women, through the menses. The skin and kidneys are the body's preferred channels for eliminating toxins from the blood. Thus, skin eruptive diseases and urinary problems are signs that the blood needs cleansing and herbs that help clear up these toxins by strengthening the ability of the liver and kidneys to remove them are appropriately called blood purifiers.

Single herbs that are considered blood purifiers include burdock, cleavers, dandelion, Oregon grape, pau d'arco, red clover and yellow dock. Several good blood purifying formulas include All Cell Detox, Blood Build, Enviro-Detox, Liver Balance and Liver Cleanse Formula.

These formulas can be used wherever there are skin eruptive diseases such as chicken pox, measles, acne or rashes. They can also be used for general malaise, where a person feels "yucky" but has no obvious symptoms. For acute conditions they should be taken in small doses (1-2 capsules) repeated frequently (every two or three hours). They should be taken with plenty of water to help flush irritants from the blood and lymph.

Drawing Baths to Flush Fat-Soluble Toxins

Fat-soluble toxins can also be removed from the body by drawing baths, using blood purifiers or other agents to pull fat-soluble toxins out of the oil ducts in the skin. Here's an example of how a drawing bath can help with skin eruptive diseases. When my youngest daughter, Katie, got the chicken pox, she had a few pox in her private area. She was scratching and they were getting red and sore. So, I put her in a bath of warm water and opened a two-ounce bottle of Oregon Grape Extract. I put about one ounce in the bath water and the rest I slathered liberally over her back, belly, arms and

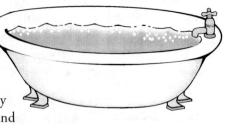

legs. I allowed her to play in the tub for 15-20 minutes, then rinsed her off and took her out. That was the end of the itching. The pox healed completely without scarring.

A variety of agents may be used in a drawing baths, but one of the best is Hydrated Bentonite, a fine clay. Clay pulls oils out of the skin (as anyone who has ever had some clay dry on you're his or her skin can attest). Put half a bottle of the Hydrated Bentonite in a warm bath and soak in it for 15-20 minutes. Then rinse off. You can also use any other fine clay used in cosmetics in drawing baths.

Blood purifiers should be taken internally, both before and after the bath. Blood purifying herbs can also be used in the bath, but one note of caution—barberry, goldenseal and yellow dock all contain a yellow dye which can color the skin. It wears off rather quickly, however.

Drawing baths will help take stress off of the liver quickly, while other internal methods of detoxification help cleanse the liver and improve its function.

In the next chapter we'll talk about the kidneys and sweat glands and how to flush water-soluble toxins out of the body.

Chapter Ten

Flushing the Body's Fluids

The colon is the primary organ for eliminating solid waste from the body, and the liver, gallbladder and sweat glands help eliminate fat-soluble toxins. Water-soluble toxins, however, are eliminated primarily through the kidneys and the sweat glands. While a general cleansing program usually contains herbs that help to flush these fluid-cleansing systems, sometimes it's important to work directly with the kidneys and sweat glands to more effectively cleanse the fluids of the body.

Our bodies are composed of up to 60% water, and the urinary system plays the primary role in managing this water. This makes the kidneys, which process water-soluble wastes, especially vital to our overall health. Even the liver (which processes fat-soluble wastes) is dependent on the kidneys because some of its detoxification processes convert fat-soluble toxins into water-soluble toxins, which must then be eliminated with the urine through the kidneys and bladder.

Our two kidneys, each the size of a large fist, are carefully protected between the spine and other abdominal organs. Although only one kidney is required, we are provided with a "spare." They are connected to the circulatory system with generous artery and vein connections. Inside each kidney there are about a million filter structures called nephrons. (Thus, kidney inflammation is called "nephritis.")

But the kidneys are much more than filters. By selectively reabsorbing water, mineral salts and glucose back into the blood stream, the kidneys help control the circulating levels of these substances. Too much water can produce high blood pressure or water retention. Too little water can cause fainting or dehydration. The circulating salts of electrolyte minerals (calcium, magnesium, sodium and potassium) are needed continuously by every cell in the body. This is so vital that these minerals will be taken out of storage in bones (including teeth) if needed to maintain balanced amounts in the blood.

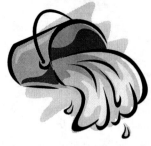

The Importance of Water

The most important key to the healthy function of this entire system is to drink plenty of clean water. In fact, water is the most important "medicine" our body needs when we are ill. This medicine is more important than any herb or supplement because without it, the body can't properly flush irritants. We've all heard the adage, "Rest in bed and drink plenty of fluids." It is good advice.

All of our eliminative channels need water to work properly. Without water, the stool becomes hard and the body gets constipated. Without water, the body can't flush toxins through the sweat glands in the skin. Water is also vital in creating a healthy flow of mucus to keep the respiratory system clear of debris. Most of all, water is vital to the function of the kidneys. The kidneys can't flush irritants from our body properly if the body is even partially dehydrated and, when one is sick, the kidneys need extra fluids to do their job.

Sometimes when people have fluid retention in their tissues, they reduce the amount of water they are drinking thinking this will help. It doesn't. The tissues are retaining fluid because of toxins and water will help to flush these toxins from the body and reduce fluid retention in the tissues.

So, be sure to drink plenty of pure water whenever you are fighting any kind of illness. I recommend drinking water purified by both reverse osmosis and carbon filtration, if possible. You may even want to invest in a reverse osmosis water treatment appliance for your home. I own a Nature's Spring unit, and it is one of the best investments in my health that I ever made.

If you have pure water available, you'll find that your body will actually start to crave it. So, having a reverse osmosis unit can actually save you money because you'll drink less juice, soda and other expensive beverages, because you'll want to quench your thirst with the real thing—pure water.

Acid/Alkaline Balance

One of the most important functions of the kidneys is to flush the acid wastes out of the blood and lymph that are the by-product of cellular energy production. If not removed by the kidneys, these acids will irritate tissues and increase inflammation. The body will seek to neutralize them by "borrowing" alkalizing minerals from various tissues. It will first borrow potassium and magnesium from muscle tissues, which causes muscle to become stiff and achy and start cramping. When supplies of these minerals run low it will borrow calcium from bones, which results in osteoporosis and joint deterioration. High levels of free calcium in the blood (there to try to neutralize excess acidity) will contribute to the development of calcifications and bone spurs, and foster the development of kidney stones.

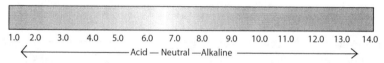

| 1.0 | 2.0 | 3.0 | 4.0 | 5.0 | 6.0 | 7.0 | 8.0 | 9.0 | 10.0 | 11.0 | 12.0 | 13.0 | 14.0 |

$\longleftarrow$ ———————— Acid — Neutral —Alkaline ———————— $\longrightarrow$

<u>Testing Your pH</u>

Most people in modern society are over acid, although occasionally you will find someone who is over alkaline. You can test your pH by obtaining some pH testing strips. Check the pH of your urine by dipping the strip in a sample of urine, preferably from the first urination in the morning. You should also test the pH of your saliva by dipping a pH test strip in a sample of your saliva. (Again, it's best to do this first thing in the morning, before breakfast.) You can also test again later in the day.

On average, the pH of your saliva should be between 6.0 and 7.0, with 6.4 to 6.6 being ideal. The pH of the urine can vary more widely, but on average should be between about 5.5 to 7.0. The saliva tests the pH of your lymphatic fluid and tells you what is happening in the tissues, while the pH of the urine tests what the body is dumping. Since the kidneys are supposed to dump acid, it is normal for the pH of the urine to be more acid than the pH of the saliva.

If you are consistently running too acid (as most people are) you will want to alkalize the body. Factors which contribute to over-acidity and place an undue burden on the kidneys include poor digestion, lack of oxygen, stress and diet. Let's examine each of these factors briefly.

Digestion and pH

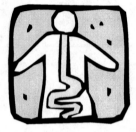

Although there are many tables claiming various foods are acid- or alkaline-forming in the body, the truth is that any food we don't digest properly creates acid waste. Hence, you can eat the best food on the planet and will still be over acid if you are lacking in digestive secretions. So, the first thing we need to do to maintain balanced pH is to maintain good digestion.

With the high percentage of cooked and processed foods in our diet, almost everyone needs to take enzyme supplements. The best choices for long-term use are the plant-enzyme products, especially Proactazyme Plus and Protease Plus. Most people need 2-4 capsules of Proactazyme with each meal of cooked food. If you have problems with protein digestion, you should also add 1-3 Protease Plus with any meal that contains a heavy protein. For problems with fat digestion add 1-2 Hi Lipase to any meal high in fat.

Oddly enough, a lack of hydrochloric acid in the stomach also contributes to acid pH. So, Protein Digestive Aid (PDA), which supplies hydrochloric acid, may be needed by some people, particularly A blood types, when eating meat or animal protein of any kind. Food Digestive Enzymes contains both hydrochloric acid and enzymes to help break food down.

Oxygen and pH

It takes oxygen to burn the nutrients we eat to create energy for our bodies. When the blood isn't carrying enough oxygen to the tissues, this contributes to the creation of more acid waste. Deep breathing therefore, can help to alkalize the body. Likewise, supplements that increase the oxygen-carrying capacity of the blood will also help.

Liquid Chlorophyll is one of the best supplements we have for increasing the oxygen supply in the blood. It appears to work by decreasing agglutination (where the red blood cells clump together, decreasing their oxygen-carrying surface). Agglutination can also be decreased by following the principles found in the books *Live Right For Your Type* and *Eat Right For Your Type* by Peter D'Adamo.

Stress and pH

We have two branches in our nervous system, the sympathetic and the parasympathetic. The sympathetic nervous system is associated with stress because it becomes very active under the influence of the adrenal glands when we are scared or upset. The sympathetic nervous system drives an acid reaction in the body that increases both tension and activity. In contrast, the parasympathetic nervous system drives a more alkaline nervous system reaction, which relaxes us. Hence, one's pH can be over acid from stress alone.

Deep breathing and relaxation exercises can help to reduce stress, but who has time for that? (That's the point, of course, we need to <u>make</u> time for relaxation, we'll never <u>find</u> it.) We can also take supplements that help reduce stress. Adaptagens are particularly useful at reducing stress responses in the body. Eleuthero (Siberian Ginseng), Chinese Mineral Chi Tonic and Nervous Fatigue Formula (HS-C) are three excellent adaptagenic products. Nervine herbs such as Stress-J (STR-J) or Herbal Sleep (HVP) can also help. Many people find also Nutri-Calm helps them keep from getting too wound up. If you suspect that stress is contributing to your pH imbalance, try a few of these products for a week and see if it helps.

Acid and Alkaline Forming Foods

Many people get confused about what foods are acid-forming and what foods are alkaline-forming in the body. First, let's get it perfectly clear that the pH of the food itself does not determine whether a food will make the body more acid or more alkaline. For example, lemons are very acidic, but they have an alkalizing effect on the body. Meat, on the other hand, is very alkaline, but it has an acidifying effect on the body.

Without going into tiresome and boring details, it essentially boils down to this—most fruits and vegetables tend to be alkalizing because they are easy to digest and high in alkaline minerals, while most grains, legumes, nuts and protein foods (dairy, eggs, meat, fish, etc.) tend to be acidifying because they are more difficult to digest and are higher in acidic minerals. This is one reason juice fasting can be so effective. It rapidly alkalizes the body and helps the kidneys flush excess acid from the tissues. To help you balance pH, Tree of Light Publishing produces *pH, Blood Type and Nutrition charts* which identify acid- and alkaline-forming foods, as well as foods which cause agglutination for each blood type.

Diuretics

If the kidneys are sluggish, they may also need a little boost from some herbal remedies called diuretics. Diuretics often work best when taken as teas, but they can also be beneficial in capsules or tinctures as long as they are taken with ample amounts of water. Here are a few of the herbs that have a diuretic effect: asparagus, buchu, celery, cleavers, cornsilk, dandelion, juniper, goldenrod, gravel root, horsetail, hydrangea, marshmallow, nettles, parsley, uva ursi and watermelon seed. The Chinese Kidney Activator is an excellent diuretic formula.

A very simple, but effective way to cleanse the fluids of the body is to mix 1 teaspoon of Lymphatic Drainage Formula in a quart of purified (Nature's Spring) water. Sip this mixture throughout the day to help flush fluid and acid waste out of the body's tissues. If there is any fluid retention, add the Chinese Kidney Activator formula and don't be shy about the amounts. You can take 2-3 capsules 3-4 times daily in order to get the full diuretic effect.

If you have problems with frequent urinary tract infections, you may also benefit from taking Cranberry/Buchu on a regular basis. Cranberry helps to prevent urinary tract infections when taken regularly and buchu is an excellent diuretic. When suffering from an acute urinary tract infection, you should add goldenseal/echinacea and/or uva ursi to the program to help fight the infection.

Urinary formulas should always be used with plenty of water to help flush irritants through the kidneys. It also helps to eat more alkalizing foods (fruits and vegetables) and avoid more acid forming foods (meats, grains and dairy) when trying to cleanse the urinary tract.

Kidney and Bladder Stones

When calcium becomes too concentrated in the urine, it can form kidney stones. Excess free calcium in the blood (free calcium is calcium that is not bound to fats [lipids] or proteins) will also contribute to kidney stones and calcification of tissues. Kidney stones can be extremely painful to pass. Herbs that dissolve kidney stones are called lithotroptics.

Many people have successfully passed kidney stones by taking the juice of four lemons in about one gallon of pure water and drinking this in a twelve-hour period with no other foods. It also helps to take hydrangea (2 capsules every 2 hours) and marshmallow (2 capsules every 2 hours). Magnesium can be helpful; use about one tablet every 2-4 hours. Lobelia can also be taken to ease pain and relax the urinary passages. Kidney stones can be serious. It is wise to consult with a physician.

Eating plenty of fresh fruits and vegetables and avoiding large quantities of meat and dairy foods can help prevent kidney stones from forming. Also, avoid taking a lot of calcium supplements, particularly calcium that is not balanced with other minerals (especially magnesium). Drinking lots of pure water, instead of other beverages, is also essential.

The Sweat Glands

Just like the oil ducts can eliminate fat-soluble toxins when the liver is overloaded, the sweat glands can be used as a back-up system for removing water-soluble toxins the kidneys can't handle. In fact, the skin has been called the third kidney by many natural healers.

The more toxins being eliminated through the skin, the more the perspiration will develop an off odor. Stinky feet, smelly underarms, etc. aren't necessarily the natural result of sweating. Rather, they are signs of a toxic body and the need to cleanse the colon, liver and kidneys. Once the body has been cleared of toxins, the perspiration odor will not be as strong.

When the sweat glands aren't working properly, it places a greater burden on the kidneys. Unfortunately, many people are plugging up their sweat glands by the use of antiperspirant deodorants. This practice closes off this channel of elimination and backs up toxins into the lymph nodes in the chest area. It also backs up toxins into the breast area.

Fortunately, body odor can be reduced by taking liquid chlorophyll internally and by using Nature's Fresh topically along with some of your favorite essential oils. The essential oils inhibit the bacteria that break toxins down and release odors. Nature's Fresh enzymatically breaks down odors and neutralizes them.

The skin is the largest organ of elimination, so enhancing elimination through the skin is usually a key factor in overcoming acute or chronic illness. This can be done via exercise and by using sweat-enhancing herbs, which are known as sudorifics or diaphoretics. These herbs enhance perspiration by moving the blood to the surface of the skin and helping to open up the sweat glands to promote elimination. Sudorific herbs include blue vervain, boneset, capsicum, chamomile, catnip, ginger, horseradish, peppermint and my favorite—yarrow. Sudorific herbs work best when taken as warm teas, or tinctures or extracts taken with warm water.

HCP-X is a great sudorific formula. It should be made into a tea by emptying the contents of 2 or 3 capsules into a cup and covering with boiling water. Steep for 3-5 minutes, strain and drink. Yarrow tea with peppermint is another great sudorific blend.

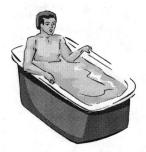

Sweat Baths

Many people in temperate climates the world over have used sweating both to prevent and treat disease. Scandinavians built saunas; Native Americans built sweat lodges. The pioneer herbalist Samuel Thomson would wrap a person sitting in a chair in blankets and place a hot stone in a pail at his feet. By pouring water into the pail, the steam would come up under the blankets until the patient started to perspire.

With modern hot running water and bathtubs, inducing perspiration to clear toxins isn't that difficult. Start by drinking plenty of water or herbal tea made from any of the previously mentioned sudorific herbs or formulas.

After drinking the tea, draw a bath as hot as can be comfortably tolerated. Add to the water a couple of tablespoons of ginger powder, a handful of rosemary or mint leaves or other aromatic herbs. Put the herbs in a cloth bag so the leaves don't get all over in the tub. Another, even easier, sweat bath water treatment is to put about 5-10 drops of an essential oil such as lavender, tea tree, eucalyptus, or peppermint in the bath. Dissolve the oils in a little liquid soap before putting them into the bath water so they will mix with the water and not just float on the surface. You can also add one to two cups of Epsom salts. (This is particularly helpful for relaxing the nerves and easing sore muscles.)

After getting out of the bath, don't dry off. Wrap up in a cotton sheet and go to bed. Pile on the blankets and allow the sweat to come freely. It's fine to fall asleep. When done, take a cool shower to cleanse the skin and close your pores. Don't allow chilling during the process.

With small children, don't put them into a really hot bath. Use a warm bath, and gently wash the child's body down with some natural soap (such as Sunshine Concentrate) and a wash cloth to make certain the pores are open. Adding just a small amount of lavender essential oil or tea tree essential oil to the bath, or using a natural soap, such as castile, will help to stimulate the circulation and draw the blood to the extremities.

I have found sweat baths to be helpful for all types of acute ailments, especially colds, fevers, flu, sinus congestion, rashes and earaches. Sweat baths are not recommended for people who are infirm, elderly or have heart conditions.

Chapter Eleven

Tissue and Lymph Cleansing

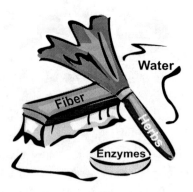

Which do you think would be a better breeding ground for mosquitoes—a bubbling, mountain brook or a pool of stagnant swamp water? We all recognize that the stagnant water is a better breeding ground for mosquitoes than a fast moving mountain stream. In other words, we all recognize that habitat or terrain is a factor in the growth of any living creature.

The same thing holds true for our bodies. Our bodies have an internal environment, which has also been called our biological terrain. Our biological terrain is based on the composition and quality of the fluids our cells live in and depend on, which include blood, lymph, gastric juices, etc. When these fluids are in proper balance, our cells prosper. When they are out of balance, not only do our own cells fail to thrive, they also create an environment conducive to the growth of unhealthy things such as fungi, bacteria, viruses, parasites or cancer cells.

Biological terrain is not a new concept, but it is one that is largely overlooked in our "germ" focused society. We tend to believe that avoiding or killing microorganisms is the only way to prevent disease. We fail to realize that before disease organisms can get a foothold, the body must provide an environment that is favorable to their growth. If the biological terrain is healthy, then disease "germs" do not have the proper conditions available for their growth. This is a major factor in a body's resistance to any illness.

In 1983, I had the opportunity to work with Dr. C. Samuel West at his International Academy of Lymphology. Dr. West was a dynamic crusader who was out to spread the word about the "gospel"

84

of lymphology. His classes were practically revival meetings dedicated to spreading the "good word" about healing the body via the lymphatic system. He is best-known for his promotion of lymphasing, or rebound exercise, on a mini-trampoline. While I never picked up Dr. West's practically religious fervor over lymphology, I did learn how important the lymphatics were to internal cleanliness and other health knowledge that has really helped my work as a natural healer.

(Speech bubble: All I need is food, water, oxygen, warmth and a clean environment!)

Each cell in the body is a miniature energy generating plant. What is happening on the macro level in the body is simply a mirror of what is happening at the cellular level. Just as we eat food, breathe oxygen, produce energy and eliminate waste, so does each cell. The cells absorb oxygen and nutrients through the cell membranes. Inside tiny energy producing factories, called mitochondria, the cells produce ATP to fuel cellular functions. Waste materials are then pumped back through the cell membrane into the surrounding environment.

The purpose of the circulatory and lymphatic systems is to provide a clean, oxygen- and nutrient-laden environment around each cell. This healthy environment is analogous to our fast-moving, bubbling mountain brook. It is the healthy terrain we all want, and it works as follows.

Fluid balance is regulated by means of osmotic pressure. In the blood stream, large molecules of three different proteins (albumin, globulin and fibrinogen) attract water and prevent it from leaking out of the pores in the blood vessels. Under normal conditions these proteins are too large to leave the circulatory system, but the pressure in the arterial end of the capillaries is great enough to force some of these proteins, albumin in particular, through the membranes and into the tissue spaces. With this protein comes some of the plasma (the fluid portion of the blood) which carries with it dissolved nutrients and oxygen.

Once this plasma has left the blood stream, it is called lymph. Lymph bathes every cell in the body. It is the great internal ocean in which all of our cells live. These lymphatic fluids are the biological terrain or internal environment of our body. The cells draw their nourishment from this lymphatic ocean and release their waste products back into it. This is why the lymphatic fluid must be kept constantly flowing. Fresh, nutrient-laden lymph fluid must be brought in as toxin-laden lymph fluid must be flushed away.

If this fluid were allowed to accumulate, the internal environment would become swampy, resulting in decreased oxygen and nutrients to the cells and increased retention of toxic waste. So removal of this protein and fluid is vital to cellular health, and that is where the lymphatics come into play.

The only way for this fluid and albumin to return to the blood stream is via the lymphatics. The lymphatic system is the other half of our circulatory system. It may help to think of the circulatory system as the water pipes that bring fresh water to your home and the lymphatic system as the sewer or septic system that drains away the waste water. This analogy can also be helpful in understanding that the blood is pumped through the vessels under pressure, just like your water supply is pressurized. The lymphatic system, however, does not have a pump. It is a passive, non-pressurized system, like your drain pipes.

How the Lymphatics Work

The lymphatics originate in the tissue spaces with tiny lymphatic capillaries which then drain into small lymphatic vessels. These in turn join together into larger lymphatic ducts. We might compare this to a watershed on a mountain range. The lymphatic capillaries are like numerous small springs scattered over a mountainside. These feed into small streams, which merge and flow into larger streams until they join into one big river.

The lymphatic "river" is the thoracic duct, located in our upper chest. Most lymphatic fluid drains into this duct, which empties its contents into the blood stream at the subclavian vein at the base of the neck. The remainder of the lymph drains into a smaller duct on the opposite side of the body.

Like the watershed or the sewer system, the water in the lymphatic stream does not go "uphill" against the current. The lymphatics flow in one direction, away from the tissues and back to the chest and bloodstream. The flow in this passive system is created by a combination of muscular activity, tissue compression, deep breathing, elasticity of the lymphatic vessels and one-way check valves. The one-way valves ensure that movement is always forward and not backward.

Deep breathing greatly increases lymphatic flow because it pumps the thoracic duct. However, movement of the body is the most powerful lymphatic pumping mechanism. Exercise increases lymph flow as much as five to fifteen times.

Understanding the passive movement in the lymphatic system explains why we feel a little stiff and sore after a prolonged period of sitting. Lack of movement slows lymphatic flow, which causes albumin and fluid to accumulate in the spaces around our cells. This diminishes oxygen and nutrient exchange, so the cells begin to complain by sending mild pain signals.

How do we respond to this? We may feel like stretching, yawning or rubbing the part that is sore. All of these activities pump lymphatic fluid, thereby diminishing fluid buildup around the cells and increasing oxygen and nutrient exchange. As a result, the cells quit complaining.

Understanding Tissue Damage

Now, let's examine the conditions that exist when tissues get hurt. Every time we damage tissues (whether we bump them, cut them, scrape them, burn them, expose them to some poisonous substance, starve them, etc.), they respond in the same way. The cellular response to damage is a process called inflammation.

Damaged cells release chemicals into the fluid surrounding the cells. One of the substances that escapes from the damaged cells is called histamine; another is bradykinin. Histamine and bradykinin cause the capillary pores to enlarge, which allows the blood proteins to escape into the tissue spaces. Since these proteins attract water, they draw large amounts of fluid into the tissue spaces. This creates swelling.

We've all seen this happen. We've bumped our head or been bitten or stung by an insect and watched the area around the injury swell. The swelling is due to the plasma proteins leaking into the spaces around the cells (interstitial spaces) and drawing fluid out of the bloodstream.

One of the proteins that leaves the blood stream is fibrinogen. This large protein is responsible for blood clots. Under normal conditions, the electrical fields surrounding the cells keep fibrinogen and the other plasma proteins in suspension. However, at the site of an injury, as cells begin to suffer a loss of oxygen and nutrients, cellular energy diminishes. This causes fibrinogen and the other proteins to clump together. In a cut, this stops the bleeding by creating a mesh that catches red blood cells to form a blood clot. In the interstitial spaces, this clotting of protein causes fluid to accumulate around the cells, which turns the normal biological terrain into a swamp. Oxygen and nutrient exchange diminishes and waste accumulates.

The same conditions that occur when we have been sitting too long have just been created on a massive scale, so our cells start complaining loudly. We experience that complaining as pain. Pain is the distress call of our tissues. When excess fluid accumulates in the tissue spaces the cells are "drowning" in fluid and waste and calling for us to throw them a life preserver.

When we understand that pain is generally a signal that there is a lack of oxygen and an increase in toxicity in the tissues spaces, we know what we need to do to answer the distress call. If we can restore the normal circulation of blood and lymph, we can restore oxygen supply to the tissues and drain away waste, thus removing the CAUSE of the pain.

Unfortunately, most people are not concerned about dealing with the cause of the pain. They just want to remove the effect, i.e., make their cells quit complaining. That's why pain killers are so popular. Pain killers work by interfering with the signals our cells relay to the brain that there is a problem. This lets us pretend that nothing is wrong.

Pain is a Warning Signal

Think of pain as a warning light in your car telling you that something is wrong with the engine. That blinking "check engine soon" light is annoying us and we're just too busy to go the mechanic to have the car checked out. So, to solve our problem we cut the wires—no more annoying light.

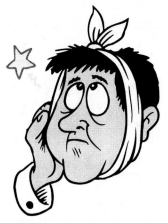

Of course, anyone with half a brain can see that this wouldn't solve our engine problem and, by ignoring the early warning signs that something is wrong, we're setting ourselves up for an even worse problem down the road. Still, that's what many of us do with our bodies. We've been trained to assume that headaches, stomachaches, muscle pains, stiff necks, etc. are just natural parts of life, so we take pain killers so we can live with them.

But the body doesn't usually complain without good reason. Pain is telling us that tissues are being damaged and we should be concerned and ask ourselves, "What is damaging my body?" It is almost like we are touching a hot stove over and over again and getting burned again and again and we are being told, "It is natural to get burned, an unavoidable part of life. Just take this pain killer for it and do your best to live with it." But we don't have to "live with it." We just have to figure out what is causing the damage and stop doing it.

If the inflammation wasn't caused by physical trauma (i.e., a physical or mechanical injury), then the cause is most likely toxins and that means we need to cleanse the body. But, cleansing isn't limited to opening the body's eliminative channels. Cells and tissues need to be cleansed, too, and this involves helping the mechanisms that produce energy to "pump" toxins out of cells and increase lymphatic drainage to carry them away.

Obviously, exercise or some form of physical activity is required to pump lymphatic fluid. It isn't going to happen if you sit at your desk and take some supplements. You should practice deep breathing and walk or at least stretch and move about regularly to keep lymph flowing properly. Gentle bouncing on a rebounder or mini-trampoline is one of the most effective lymph moving exercises you can perform, but any kind of physical activity is better than none.

Sometimes certain herbs or nutrients are needed to help cells detoxify and lymph to move more freely. Cellular Energy is a formula that contains nutrients needed in the mitochondria of the cell for energy production. It will help cells pump toxins out of the cell and into the surrounding lymphatic fluid more efficiently. However, this isn't going to be enough if the lymphatics are stagnant.

If you are bloated, overweight, lethargic or in any kind of chronic pain, then you have some degree of lymphatic stagnation. Besides moving, here is a program you can use to increase lymphatic drainage and improve cellular detoxification.

- 1 capsule Cellular Energy three times daily

- 2-3 capsules of Chinese Kidney Activator three times daily

- 1 capsule Lymphomax three times daily

- Mix the following in a quart of purified water and sip frequently throughout the day:

  - 1/2-1 teaspoon Lymphatic Drainage Formula

  - 1/2-1 teaspoon Red Clover Blend

Enzyme Systems and Detoxification

The body uses numerous enzymes to facilitate the process of internal detoxification. These enzyme systems alter toxins so they can be more easily excreted from the body. There are two steps to this process. Phase one detoxification involves about 50 different enzymes which electrically charge toxins (adding or eliminating electrons) in preparation for phase two detoxification. Some toxins do not require phase one processing and are already electrically charged, so they can go directly to phase two.

Phase two detoxification involves enzymes that add chemical groups to toxins (a process called conjugation). The conjugates (or chemical groups which are added to the molecules) include sugars, amino acids, glutathione, methionine, sulfur and acetyl Co-A. to make them water soluble so they can be excreted from the body. Most are eliminated through the kidneys, but molecules of high molecular weight are excreted through bile.

Most of the time phase 1 detoxification results in creating a less toxic substance, but some toxins become more toxic after phase one alteration. If phase two detoxification isn't strong, the person may become sicker as a result of these altered toxins. Since amino acids are needed for phase two detoxification, protein deficiency may inhibit this second phase of detoxification.

Because nutrients are needed to activate both phase one and phase two enzyme systems, people who are severely depleted nutritionally can't cleanse effectively. This is why I have repeated taught that people who are in a very weak and debilitied state should go on a building program before they attempt a cleanse. It is necessary to build up their nutrient reserves before the tissues will be able to effectively detoxify.

Nutrtional Requirements for Internal Detoxification

Phase 1 Detoxification	Phase 2 Detoxification
• Beta-carotene	• Vitamins:
• Vitamins:	– Folic Acid
– B1	– B-Complex
– C	– C
– E	• Minerals:
• Minerals:	– Germanium
– Copper	– Magnesium
– Iron	– Manganese
– Magnesium	– Molybdenum
– Manganese	– Selenium
– Molybdenum	– Sulfur
– Sulfur	– Zinc
– Zinc	• Amino Acids
• Choline	– Cysteine
• Fatty Acids	– Glycine
• Lecithin	– L-glutathione
• Methionine	– Taurine
	• N-acetyl-cysteine

See the table above to learn the nutrients needed for both phases of detoxification.

Also remember that tissue and lymphatic cleansing won't be effective if your colon, liver and kidneys aren't working properly. If any of these major eliminative organs are "plugged up" you'll stir up toxins and release them into the blood and lymph, but the body won't be able to dispose of them. Hence, they'll make you feel sick. So, make certain your bowels are moving and your kidneys and liver are working properly if you are going to do tissue cleansing.

When Cleansing Isn't a Good Idea

Cleansing isn't for everyone. Pregnant women and nursing mothers should not go on cleanses (although taking fiber and enzymes while pregnant or nursing is fine). People who are wasting or malnourished shouldn't be cleansed, either. If people are cold, pale, anemic, extremely weak or very thin, they need to focus on building their nutritional reserves before they try cleansing. In other words, they need to build before they cleanse. Cleansing can also be overdone.

I learned for myself how cleansing can be overdone when a midwife I know asked me to help her friend. The friend had done extensive cleansing using juice fasting and a mild food diet (only eating fruits and vegetables). She had also repeatedly used enemas and cleansing herbs. One morning she didn't feel well and asked the midwife to come over. The midwife arrived just as her friend started to experience a siezure. The overcleansed friend was taken to the hospital where blood tests revealed she had washed a large percentage of the electrolytes (salts of sodium, potassium, calcium and magnesium) from her body.

When I saw the lady she was nothing but skin and bones. My first thought was, "You've got nothing left to get rid of!" I told her she didn't need to cleanse, she needed to build. I had her add whole grains and animal protein back into her diet and gave her Food Enzymes to help her break it down. She improved rapidly.

The moral of the story is to use common sense. Cleansing isn't a "cure-all," and it needs to be alternated with building therapies, which nourish the body and strengthen the organs and glands. If you are in doubt about whether you are strong enough to do a cleanse, consult with a qualified herbalist, naturopath or holistic MD for advice.

Chapter Twelve

Cleanse and Breathe Freely

As a child I was taken to the doctor and received penicillin for every cold and minor ailment. As a teenager, I was put on penicillin daily for two years straight for sinus problems and at the end of those two years my sinus problems were worse. At age 16, I had an operation for a deviated septum, but my sinuses were congested again within a few weeks of the surgery.

Finally, at age 19 I developed walking pneumonia and was in bed for two weeks while being given tetracycline and another antibiotic (ampicillin). It was only when I started seeing a chiropractor and began changing my diet that I finally started to obtain relief. Permanent relief, however, came when I did a colon cleansing program for about two months.

Frequent or chronic respiratory problems are a symptom that the lymphatic system is burdened and sluggish. This is true in the case of chronic sinus congestion, chronic post nasal drip, frequent coughing, hayfever and allergy induced asthma. There is also a host of secondary conditions that develop from this same root cause. These include sore throats, earaches, swollen lymph nodes and tonsillitis. The tonsils are lymphatic tissue and are part of our immune system. They become inflamed when the burden of irritants is so great that it overwhelms the lymphatic system in the head area and the toxins actually inflame the very system that is supposed to neutralize them. The same thing is happening to a lesser degree with swollen lymph nodes.

It is important to understand that the lymphatic system becomes congested when the colon and kidneys are overburdened or weakened. So, whenever you encounter frequent respiratory problems, especially chronic ones, you also need to improve elimination through the colon and kidneys. Allergic reactions in the intestinal tract will also increase irritation in the mucus membrane linings of the respiratory passages.

In Chinese medicine, the colon and lungs are considered part of the "metal" element. Metal is the stuff of swords and shields—weapons of defense. Our defensive, or immune, capacity is concentrated on the mucus membrane linings of the respiratory and digestive systems. They constitute our first line of immune defense in protecting the body from invasion of microorganisms or toxins.

The mucus, which coats the lining of both the digestive tract and the respiratory tract is primarily composed of lymphatic fluid. Under normal conditions, the lymphatic system is able to "dump" debris into the mucus of the colon for elimination. However, if the colon isn't emptying properly, this material will back up into the respiratory tract, which will have to handle the overload. So, just as the oil ducts handle a toxic overload from the liver and the sweat glands are the back up to the kidneys, the lungs and sinuses serve as a backup dumping ground for the lymphatics when the colon is plugged. This is why we stressed the importance of having the colon working properly before doing tissue cleansing. If the colon isn't emptying out, the lymphatic debris will have no where to go except through the lungs and sinuses.

Foods that are difficult for our body to break down will congest the lymphatic system and lead to excess mucus production. Dairy foods are common culprit. However, they are not the only foods that contribute to lymphatic congestion and it's many manifestations. Grains, especially wheat, and animal proteins, such as meat and eggs, can also be contributing factors to these conditions. Refined sugar and salt can also aggravate these conditions.

This can easily be observed by noticing how young children tend to get sick around holidays when well-meaning teachers, friends and family (including their parents) give them too many "treats." Of course, adults also are more prone to these problems when they consume large quantities of these foods, especially when their genetic make-up makes it difficult for them to digest them. This is why it is important for anyone, child or adult, who is congested to avoid dairy, grains (except rice and millet), salt, sugar, eggs, and meat.

Antibiotics and Antihistamines Aren't The Answer

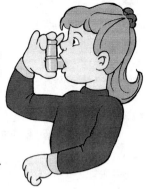

Unfortunately, when most people have respiratory congestion, they don't help the body clean itself out. Instead, the want to plug up the system further with antibiotics and antihistamines.

As a professional herbalist, I've observed children receiving frequent rounds of antibiotics. Like I was as a child, they are sickly and pale. Their eyes are dull and listless. Their immune systems are weak. Antibiotics are just adding to the toxic overload of the body. They aren't helping to remove the cause of the congestion.

Antihistamines aren't an answer either. Antihistamines "turn off the faucet" but they do so by drying up sinus secretions without addressing underlying causes. This provides temporary relief but make the problem worse in the long run. Years ago I was shown a clipping from the Wall Street Journal that reported the results of a study on antihistamines. It showed that taking antihistamines doubled the length of time it took to recover from a cold. Taking antihistamines is like trying to put a cork into one of our body's eliminative systems. It's only interfering with the efforts of our body to remove what is irritating it.

So, if these drugs aren't the solution, what is? Well, besides doing some general cleansing, there are some specific things one can do to help clean out the respiratory passages.

Excessive drainage is caused by inflammation of the sinus membranes due to the presence of some irritating substance. When the tissues are damaged by irritants, they release histamines which dilate the blood capillaries and allow excess fluid to enter the tissue spaces. In the case of sinus problems, these excess fluids drain out onto the surface of the mucus membranes, which helps to flush the irritants away. Sinus drainage, watery eyes, sneezing, post-nasal drip and coughing are all ways of flushing irritants through the respiratory system. And, just as nausea, vomiting and diarrhea can be thought of as a liver crisis, respiratory congestion and all of the conditions that accompany it can be thought of as a lymphatic crisis. The key is to assist, rather than fight the process.

Sinus Drainage

Sinus drainage begins with the discharge of a thin, watery mucus, which represents the attempt of the tissues to wash away irritating toxins. The fact that this watery mucus often burns (or inflames) the upper part of the lip demonstrates it's toxic nature. We do not want to stop the flow of this mucus because we want the body to be able to flush these irritants, so what we need are remedies that will enhance, not diminish, this drainage. The pungent aromatic herbs are extremely beneficial here.

Think of a time when you ate something that was really spicy. Changes are, your face got flushed, your eyes started to water and your nose started to run. This is exactly the effect we need in these early stages of a cold or respiratory infection. Any spicy herbs, consumed with lots of water, can work wonders in the early stages of a sinus drainage. These include capsicum, garlic, ginger, horseradish, mustard and thyme.

I've "burned off" many a cold in its very early stages by using these spicy herbs. One of my favorite remedies for the early stages of a cold is hot tomato soup with capsicum or cayenne pepper added to it. I've also used fresh horseradish, hot Chinese mustard and fresh apple juice with lemon and a little bit of fresh ginger juice to successfully eliminate a cold in the very early stages. Always use these herbs with plenty of fluids as the body needs water to continue producing this thin, watery mucus.

My favorite formula for clearing congestion is ALJ. The key is to take large quantities at frequent intervals, such as 2-4 capsules every 2 hours with plenty of water. For infection in the lungs I add 1 capsule of High Potency Garlic every 4 hours. This will help to loosen the mucus so the body can sneeze out, cough out or otherwise expel whatever is irritating the lungs.

Remember that as soon as the body has successfully discharged whatever was irritating it, the symptoms will cease and you will start to feel better. If, however, the body is unable to flush the irritation in these early stages, then a more chronic congestion settles in. As the body loses moisture and the tissues become progressively weakened by the irritants, the mucus thickens to become white and harder to eliminate. Eventually, as infection and heat settle in, the mucus becomes discolored.

In these later stages of sinus drainage, another group of herbs is needed to help thin the mucus and allow the body to clear the congestion. These herbs are called decongestants. ALJ is a decongestant, but I like to use either Fenugreek & Thyme and Goldenseal & Echinacea along with AL-J for the later stages of a cold or congestion. Fenugreek & Thyme is good for sinus congestion and sinus headaches, while Goldenseal & Echinacea is better for sinus infection. These herbs, again taken at regular intervals with plenty of water, will thin the mucus and help to flush the mucus membranes, so the body can more easily clear the irritation.

Coughing and Sneezing

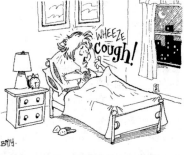

Both our sinuses and our lungs are coated with tiny hair-like projections called cilia. As we breath, dust particles and other debris enter our respiratory passages. They become trapped in the thin layer of mucus that coats these membranes. The cilia sweep this mucus, and the debris it has trapped, to the esophagus so it can be swallowed and eliminated from out body. Post-nasal drip is caused by excessive mucus being swept out of the sinuses to the back of the throat. When we "clear our throat" we are moving excess mucus out of the bronchials and into the esophagus.

Sometimes, the mucus gets too thick for the cilia to sweep it along. It gets "stuck" so to speak. This causes the cilia to become irritated and we have a nervous reflex action that causes us to cough or sneeze the try to break up the thick mucus. Over-the-counter cough medications contain cough suppressants, medications that interfere with the nervous system so that the cough reflex is suppressed. While this may help you get some sleep, it does nothing to help the body remove the cause of the irritation.

There is a class of herbs, however, that can help the body expel irritants trapped in the lungs or sinuses. The are called expectorants because of their ability to help expectorate mucus. All of the herbs previously mentioned can act as expectorants, but here are some addition remedies that may be helpful. Lobelia is very good for spastic coughs. It relaxes muscle spasms to make it easier to expel mucus. Marshmallow and Fenugreek or Licorice root can be helpful for dry coughs because they help to hydrate lung tissue when taken with lots of water.

Allergic Reactions

Allergic reactions to pollen, dust, molds, pet dander and other environmental allergens are signs of an overtaxed immune system and a generally toxic condition in the body. Following many of the cleansing procedures listed in this book, as well as improving one's diet can go a long way towards reducing allergic reactions.

Respiratory allergies occur because of hypersensitive immune reactions on the mucus membranes. An allergen comes in contact with an antibody—a chemical produced by the body to sequester or neutralize an offending substance. These reactions take place on specialized cells called mast cells. When the immune system is over reactive, these mast cells burst, releasing (you guessed it) histamine and bradykinin, which trigger the inflammatory response.

So, allergies are nothing more than another inflammatory reaction to an irritant. The inflammation causes excess mucus production to try to flush the irritant. If other eliminative chimneys, such as the colon, liver and kidneys, are functioning properly these reactions are not as severe.

There are a number of herbs that help to maintain tissue integrity and inhibit mast cells from bursting to trigger these inflammatory reactions. These herbs are natural antihistamines and mast cell stabilizers. ALJ has some anti-allergenic effect, but the best formula is Hista-Block.

Massage for Congestion

As mentioned, many respiratory problems start with sluggish lymphatic drainage. Increasing lymphatic drainage using the physical movement and some of the remedies we mentioned in the last chapter can be very helpful for cleaning out respiratory congestion. Directly massaging the chest with some essential oils diluted in a massage oil is also very helpful. Oils that are good for respiratory congestion include eucalyptus, lavender, rosemary, thyme and tea tree oil.

Dilute these essential oils in olive oil (or another fixed oil) by adding one part of essential oils for 10 parts of oil. (In other words, one drop of essential oil for every ten drops of oil.) For babies and toddlers you can dilute the essential oils even more, about one part essential oil to twenty parts olive oil.

I've rubbed these mixtures onto the chest and throat many times to reduce lymphatic congestion and ease respiratory problems. In particular, these oils should be massaged into swollen lymph nodes in the neck and chest.

Chapter Thirteen

Cleaning the Pipes

The blood stream is the river of life, the source of life-giving oxygen and nutrients for every cell in the body. Unfortunately, cardiovascular disease has become the number one cause of death in civilized countries.

Atherosclerosis—hardening of the arteries—is caused by the arterial walls hardening and thickening from deposits of plaque, which causes a narrowing of the arteries. Oxidized cholesterol (LDL cholesterol that has combined with unstable oxygen molecules) coats the damaged arteries, increasing the condition and bringing risk of heart attack and stroke. Heart attacks, alone, are responsible for over 550,000 deaths in the United States every year!

Over 60 million Americans suffer from some form of heart disease, resulting in over $56 billion a year in medical costs for treatment of these conditions. Heart bypass surgeries, angioplasties (surgical altering of blood vessels), limb amputations caused by damage to extremities due to shutdown circulation and cholesterol-lowering drugs are just a part of the scene.

There is a natural approach that offers a way to deal with and help to prevent these and other conditions safely, effectively, and at an incredibly reduced cost in both dollars and human suffering— Chelation. Pronounced key-LAY-shun, this odd word originally comes from Greek roots. "Chele" means "to claw" or "to bind or grab." When we use it in the word chelation, we are talking about "clawing," "grabbing" or otherwise binding toxins, heavy metals, metabolic wastes and unhealthy buildup in the circulatory system. This allows them to be taken out of the bloodstream so they can be flushed from the body.

Intravenous chelation therapy with EDTA (a synthetic amino acid that binds up or "chelates" heavy metals), has been shown to be safe and effective in reversing atherosclerosis (hardening of the arteries), preventing heart attacks and strokes, improving circulation and overall health, and can be used as an alternative to bypass surgery and angioplasty. It takes a series of visits to a medical doctor (MD), or licensed naturopathic medical doctor (NMD), who practices chelation therapy for intravenous treatments, to accomplish these results.

Unfortunately, even with the overwhelming positive results reported by doctors who use chelation therapy, the FDA and AMA still refuse to endorse this form of medical treatment. There are those who suggest that this stand is more motivated by the financial agendas of large pharmaceutical companies (who cannot make money on a commonly available food additive like ETDA), rather than a true concern for the health care needs of the hundreds of thousands of people who could benefit from the therapy.

About Chelation Therapy

Brought to the United States in 1948, chelation therapy was developed in Germany in the early 1930s. Besides clearing the arteries of plaque that has built up in the arteries, chelation therapy is currently used around the world for treatment of heavy metal toxicity. Heavy metals are any mineral such as mercury, lead, arsenic, aluminum, nickel, cadmium and others that accumulate in fat cells, the central nervous system and other body tissues and are known to cause negative effects to health. Exposure to these and other toxic components is generally increasing in our society and environment, not decreasing, and so are the subsequent challenges to our health.

Besides being helpful for cardiovascular disease and heavy metal poisoning, intravenous chelation therapy is also reported to be effective in treatment of radiation toxicity, snake venom poisoning, irregular heartbeat, improving circulation to the extremities, and for preventing or reversing most heart and artery problems and disease. There are those in both the medical and holistic professions who feel that some forms of Alzheimer's and other auto-immune disorders can also benefit from chelation therapy.

Oral Chelation

Doctors who practice intravenous chelation are hard to come by, but there is a less expensive and easy-to-obtain alternative—oral chelation. Oral chelation uses natural, nutritional products in the home without having to step into a doctor's office or experience the harsh reactions of intravenous chelation. However, it is important to know that oral chelation is gentler and slower acting than intravenous chelation, creating less dramatic results at the outset. Unless there is a life threatening need (which should be handled by clinical health care providers, anyway), oral chelation is a wonderful option for those who wish to improve their cardiovascular health. Properly administered, oral chelation is noninvasive, quite effective, relatively inexpensive and very safe.

Here is how oral chelation works. Free radicals are unstable molecules that steal electrons from other molecules, causing harm to the body's health. What this means is that when a free radical molecule comes in contact with a stable molecule, it pulls an electron from the stable molecule, which makes the molecule unstable and chemically reactive within the body. Formerly benign and nontoxic molecules then become toxic to the body.

Many nutritionally based substances are free radical 'scavengers'. These free radical scavengers grab and pull toxins from the bloodstream, safeguarding health and helping the immune system do its job. This process helps the body remove arterial plaque and heavy metals from the system.

Examples of nutritional substances that act as free radical scavengers include the antioxidant nutrients vitamin C, A, E, beta carotene, selenium, coenzyme Q10, Grapine (pycnogenol), gingko biloba and garlic. Mega-Chel uses high doses of these and other substances to produce a chelation effect in the blood stream. Its thirty-five different nutritional ingredients have proven time and again to produce amazing results similar to those of intravenous chelation.

Mega-Chel Oral Chelation Program

What follows is a description of a complete oral chelation program featuring Mega-Chel. Success stories resulting from the use of the MegaChel program are legion. Many people have reported dramatic increases in blood circulation to the extremities, helping people to avoid coronary by-pass surgery and reducing their risk of heart attack and stroke. MegaChel often helps to lower blood pressure and cholesterol levels (although it may cause an increase in both of these problems in the early stages of the program). Mega Chel (in combination with other supplements) has also been reported to help heal varicose veins, senility, cold extremities, gangrene, heavy metal poisoning, calcification of tissues, macular degeneration and ulcerations in the extremities.

Remember, the MegaChel Program is designed to take several months. The older you are, the longer you need to stay on it for the fullest results of chelation in the body. This program isn't designed for instant results, but for safe and thorough results.

General Instructions

It is very important to start slowly with this program and work up as instructed. Otherwise, symptoms, such as nausea, dizziness, headaches and skin eruptions, may occur. It is also important to taper off as instructed, or fatigue and temporary nutritional deficiencies may result. It is not a good idea to do the oral chelation program if you are pregnant or nursing. This program is also not recommended for children or teenagers.

Working Up to Full Dose

For the first week, take the following with breakfast and dinner.

• 1 tablet of Mega-Chel

• 1/2 ounce of Mineral Chi Tonic or Colloidal Minerals

Each week increase the dosage of Mega-Chel by 1 tablet. Hence, the second week, take 2 tablets of Mega-Chel. Gradually increase the amount of minerals until you are taking 1 ounce in the morning and 1 ounce at night.

Full Program

A full dose of Mega-Chel is 4-6 tablets twice daily, depending on body weight. Large persons should take the full 6 tablets two times per day. Small persons should take 4 tablets two times per day. Individuals of average height and weight should find 5 tablets two times per day (for a total of 10 per day) sufficient. When you reach full dose, you will be taking the following with breakfast and dinner:

- 4-6 Mega-Chel Tablets

- 1 ounce of Colloidal Minerals or Mineral Chi Tonic

You will need to stay on this full dose for a minimum of 1 month for each ten years of your age. Thus, if you are 40 you need to stay on the full dose for at least 4 months, 6 months if you are 60, etc.

Tapering Off

It is important to taper off in a similar manner to building up. On the full program you are taking very large doses of certain vitamins and minerals, and the body gets lazy about extracting them from food.

Hence, if you quit all at once, your body may experience a sudden drop in nutrient levels until it readjusts to absorbing these vitamins and minerals from food. Taper off by reducing the amount you take by two tablets each week. After the program is complete, some people use Mega-Chel as their daily vitamin and mineral supplement by taking two tablets per day.

Cleansing Reactions

As the body removes the plaque from the walls of the arteries, the cholesterol level in the blood will temporarily rise. This is normal. The kidneys and liver will remove the calcium, cholesterol and other impurities from the body. If there are indications that these organs are weak, it may be necessary to give them extra support as follows:

For persons with kidney weakness (history of symptoms like arthritis, chronic back pain, urinary infections, etc.): 2 KB-C with each meal, or Lymphatic Drainage and Kidney Drainage in water sipped throughout the day.

For persons with liver weakness (history of high cholesterol, skin problems, digestive upset, etc.): 1 teaspoon of. LOCLO in a large glass of water or juice upon arising and before retiring, 2 Chinese Liver Balance with each meal.

Optional Supplements

You may also wish to add some of the following supplements for special problems. These are suggested full doses. You can work up gradually on taking these supplements as well.

- For heart problems: 2 HS II or 2 Hawthorn Berries with each meal

- For senility: 2 Ginkgo/Hawthorn with each meal

- For varicose veins and high risk of stroke: 2 Butcher's Broom with each meal or 1 Vari-Gone twice daily.

Chelation Diet

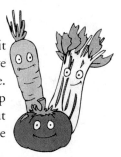

Any health recovery regime is incomplete if it doesn't address the dietary habits that may have contributed to the condition in the first place. These dietary recommendations will not only help the oral chelation program be more effective, but when adopted as a dietary lifestyle, will contribute to continuing greater health and wellbeing.

- Cut out white sugar. White sugar not only makes cavities, but wreaks havoc on blood sugar levels, brain function, vitamin and mineral absorption and overall health. A small amount of honey or raw, unrefined sugar is permissible.

- Eat whole grain cereals and breads, not white flour. Use whole grains as much as possible in cooking and unbleached flour if whole grain flour won't work for a particular recipe. Include lots of fiber in the diet. Remember that fiber absorbs the bile from the liver, which is how the body gets rid of excess cholesterol.

- Bake your potatoes and eat the skins, too. No French fries! In fact, don't eat greasy fast food at all! There are many ways to cook your potatoes without frying them.

- Reduce your table salt intake. Use sea salt or RealSalt™, not regular salt, which is filled with additives.

- Use olive oil, canola oil and safflower oil for cooking. Avoid deep frying and don't use margarine, Limit your use of butter. A good rule of thumb is that if a fat is solid at room temperature it is saturated, it saturated fats aren't good for your body in large quantites. The exception is coconut oil. Also avoid hydrogenated fats and transfatty acids.

- Avoid most dairy products. Choose to eat plain yogurt and natural, light cheeses only. Eat up to six eggs (only) per week, soft-boiled or poached; not scrambled or hard cooked.

- Eat raw, uncooked nuts and seeds. Almonds, pecans, pumpkin seeds, flax seeds and sunflower seeds are best. Stay away from salted nuts or hydrogenated peanut butter.

- Drink lots of purified water, at least 6-8 large glasses a day. It is important to do our best to avoid putting more toxic chemicals into the body. Use a Nature's Spring reverse osmosis water purifier.

- Eat lots of vegetables. specially green leafy vegetables such as chard, spinach, broccoli, cabbage; orange vegetables such as carrots, yellow squashes, pumpkin; romaine and leafy lettuces, and sprouts of all kinds. Experiment with alfalfa, radish, mung bean, wheat, lentil, and other grains and seeds. Include as much variety of vegetables in your diet as possible. This is one of the big keys to cardiovascular health. Eat vegetables lightly steamed or Oriental stir-fry style.

- Load up on antioxidants. Antioxidants help prevent inflammation, which is the underlying cause of cardiovascular disease. Fresh fruits and vegetables are your best sources of antioxidant nutrients. Supplement these with Thai-Go, Co-Q10 75 or Grapine.

Keep your pipes clean and your blood flowing freely so that all your cells will receive the oxygen and nutrients they need. The oral chelation program can also be effective in helping to eliminate heavy metals, the topic of the next chapter.

Chapter Fourteen

Heavy Metal Detoxification

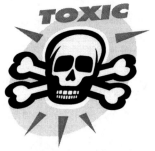

Rome may not have been built in a day, but it was destroyed by heavy metal poisoning in its water supply! The Roman aqueduct system and the plumbing of the famous baths and in the residences of the ruling class of Rome were incredible for their time, but the lead pipes in the civic water system caused neurological disorders that lead to the decadent behavior that caused the Roman Empire to collapse.

Today, heavy metals and other toxic substances in our environment are bringing about a similar decline in the mental (and physical) health of society. Learning disabilities and behavioral problems are rampant, and a new set of diseases, autoimmune disorders, have been increasing at an alarming rate. These include rheumatoid arthritis, chronic fatigue, type I diabetes, fibromyalgia, lupus, Lou Gherig's disease, myasthenia gravins and multiple sclerosis. Heavy metals and other environmental contaminants are likely a major factor.

Before we look at how to cleanse the body of these metals and toxins, let's learn a little more about heavy metals and how they get into the body.

Arsenic

It's not little old ladies like those in the play "Arsenic and Old Lace" who are causing the high levels of arsenic poisoning that we are seeing in our society. It's influences like pesticides, laundry aids, smog, cigarette smoke, table salt, seafood, and even contaminated drinking water that are the culprits.

75

As

ARSENIC

33

Symptoms of arsenic poisoning include confusion, convulsions, drowsiness and headaches. Toxic levels of arsenic can cause coma and death. Arsenic can also cause cancers. People working around pesticides, mining, and metallurgical work are at high risk of developing high levels of arsenic toxicity. In case of accidental arsenic poisoning, take charcoal tablets immediately and get medical help.

Aluminum

Al ²⁷

Aluminum isn't technically a heavy metal, but it can be toxic the same way. Symptoms are the same as Alzheimer's disease and osteoporosis. Anemia, poor calcium metabolism, forgetfulness, gastrointestinal disturbances, headaches, liver and kidney function problems, memory loss, nervousness, speech disturbances, softening of the bones, and weak, aching muscles are some symptoms of possible aluminum toxicity.

ALUMINUM 13

Aluminum is excreted through the kidneys, so it can seriously impair kidney function. When it effects the brain, it causes seizures and reduced mental faculties.

Aluminum fluoride is already one of the most abundant metallic elements in the earth's crust. It permeates our air, water and soil. Trace amounts of aluminum are essential to our health when consumed in a chelated form in foods. But when we add aluminum through our cookware, cooking utensils and many other products, we overload our bodies to dangerous levels. These toxic forms of aluminum replace the good, chelated aluminum in our bodies. Some of our everyday sources of aluminum are baking powder, toiletry items, dental amalgams, many medications (like antacids), some food items, underarm deodorants and unfiltered water.

Cadmium

Cadmium accumulates in the body, replacing zinc in the liver and kidneys. Toxic levels of cadmium may cause anemia, loss of appetite, hair loss, high blood pressure, joint soreness, dull sense of smell, and dry, scaly skin. Also, cadmium weakens the immune system by lowering the levels of T cells (white blood cells that protect the body from foreign invaders and cancer cells), can cause kidney disease and liver damage, cancer, emphysema and shortened life span. Cadmium is found in cigarette smoke, plastics, nickel-cadmium batteries, drinking water, fertilizer, fungicides, pesticides, soil, air pollution, refined grains, rice and soft drinks.

Lead

Lead is one of the most toxic metals known. It's been many years since our society was made aware of the damage that exposure to lead-based paints was doing to our health, especially to young children who suck on and chew anything they can get their hands on and their little mouths around.

When the lead reaches toxic levels in the body, it can damage the kidneys, liver, heart and nervous system. The body can't tell the difference between lead and calcium, so pregnant women, children and other people who are deficient in calcium absorb lead more easily, with children effected the most severely. Possible symptoms of lead poisoning include anxiety, arthritis, confusion, chronic fatigue, behavioral problems, juvenile delinquency, hyperactivity, learning disabilities, metallic taste in the mouth, tremors, mental disturbances, loss of memory, mental retardation, impotence, reproductive disorders, infertility, liver failure and death. It's easy to see how lead pipes contributed to the fall of the Roman Empire.

Exposure to lead can come from food that is grown near roads or factories, lead-based paint, hair products, food from lead-soldered cans, imported ceramic products (especially from Mexico and China), lead crystal glassware, ink on bread bags, batteries in cars, bone meal, insecticides, tobacco, lead pipes, and lead solder in the water pipes. If you suspect you could have lead pipes or lead solder in your water system, have the water tested.

Mercury

Mercury is even more toxic than lead. Mercury is found in our soil, water, food supply, sewage sludge, fungicides, pesticides, some grains and seeds that are treated with methyl mercury chlorine bleach (which also seeps into the food supply and contaminates our waters and fish). Also, mercury is found in many everyday products such as cosmetics, dental fillings,

109

fabric softeners, inks, tattoo ink, latex, some medications and vaccines, paints, plastics, polishes, solvents and wood preservatives.

Mercury has long been known to be one of the most toxic substances to the human body that there is. Mercury vapors carry minute and microscopic amounts into the lungs and the bloodstream where they settle into the tissues.

Broken mercury thermometers aren't the only way we can be exposed to mercury, which in its natural form is a liquid metal that should not even be touched as it can absorb directly into the skin. Remember those silver fillings that dentists put into your mouth? Well, they are really a silver/mercury amalgam! According to the World Health Organization, amalgam dental fillings are a major source of mercury exposure. These so-called 'silver fillings' contain 50% mercury, 25% silver, and 25% other materials such as copper, tin and nickel.

Minimizing Exposure to Heavy Metals

So, what can we do to protect ourselves from heavy metals? Here are a few tips.

- First, drink purified water! This is one of the most important things you can do to protect yourself and your family on an ongoing basis. A Nature's Spring reverse osmosis water treatment system is the best way to do this. I wouldn't be without one!

- Make sure your water pipes have no lead, avoid lead-based painted objects, don't store liquids in lead crystal containers.

- Buy organic food as much as possible. Pesticides and agricultural chemicals can contain heavy metals.

- Keep the chemicals in your life, especially cleaning chemicals, to a minimum.

- Avoid cooking with aluminum pans or cooking in aluminum foil with anything that is reactive with aluminum (most acid foods are).

- Insist on composite fillings from your dentist, not mercury/silver amalgams, and have existing amalgams replaced as you are able.

Fortunately, many dentists are switching to other filling materials, but many people still have these fillings in their mouths, which are constantly exposing the body to mercury poisoning, especially as the fillings deteriorate. Many people with these conditions have had their fillings removed and have had significant improvement to their health. It's important to do some heavy metal detox after amalgam filling removal.

Mercury passes through the blood-brain barrier and can cause autoimmune disorders, arthritis, blindness, candidiasis, depression, dizziness, fatigue, gum disease, hair loss, insomnia, memory loss, muscle weakness, multiple sclerosis, lateral sclerosis (ALS), Alzheimer's, Parkinson's, paralysis, lupus, food and environmental allergies, menstrual disorders, miscarriages, behavioral changes, depression, irritability, hyperactivity, allergic reactions, asthma, metallic taste in the mouth, loose teeth and more.

Heavy Metal Cleansing

Because the body is naturally exposed to small amounts of heavy metals in even natural foods, it has natural defensive mechanisms to help it eliminate these heavy metals and other toxic substances from our body. By nutritionally supporting these mechanisms, while keeping the body's channels of elimination open, one can help the body remove excess heavy metals from the system.

Glutathione and N-acetyl-cysteine

One of the principal detoxifying agents in the body is a substance called glutathione. It is an antioxidant, produced in the liver from three amino acids: cysteine, glutamic acid and glycine. Glutathione helps cells eliminate drugs and heavy metals and protects the body from damage from smoking, radiation and alcohol.

N-acetyl-cysteine (NAC) contains the amino acid cysteine, which is a building block for glutathione, a powerful antioxidant that protects tissues including the liver, respiratory and immune systems, and the eyes. Glutathione protects healthy cells from damage by heavy metals and other toxic chemicals.

L-methionine is a sulfur bearing amino acid that acts as a powerful antioxidant. It is needed in extra amounts when toxins are present in the body because it protects glutathione. It can also be converted into cysteine to help produce more glutathione.

Another nutrient that helps the body detox from heavy metals is alpha lipoic acid, a powerful antioxidant. Because it is soluble in both water and fat, it has an especially wide range of protective actions. Even more, it enhances the function of other antioxidants like vitamin C, vitamin E, and glutathione. It also helps increase energy production in the cells.

Algin and Fiber

Sodium alginate or algin is a mucilage derived from kelp. Kelp is a purifier of the oceans because the alginate in it bonds to heavy metals and other toxins to neutralize them. Sodium alginate binds to heavy metals such as lead and mercury in the intestinal tract and carries them out of body with regular bowel movements. Other fiber products such as apple pectin can also help bind heavy metals.

Heavy Metal Detox

The Heavy Metal Detox formula contains all the substances we've just mentioned—N-acytl-cysteine, l-methionine, alpha lipoic acid and sodium alginate. It also contains cilantro, an herb reported to help the body detoxify from mercury, kelp, vitamin B6, apple pectin and magnesium citrate. It is a very useful supplement for helping the body eliminate heavy metals. This formula is a potent cleanser. Do not exceed 1 capsule with a meal 2 times a day, at least in the beginning. If you develop a strong cleansing reaction (rash, diarrhea, nausea, dizziness, weakness, etc.), stop taking it for a couple of days. Do some cleansing and then restart with only 1 capsule per day.

Essential Fatty Acids

Many heavy metals (and other environmental toxins) are not water-soluble. This means the body must remove them by binding them to fats. Thus, essential fatty acids are very helpful in detoxifying from heavy metals. Daily supplementation with 1-2 Tablespoons of Flax Seed Oil (or taking Super GLA and/or Omega-3 Hi EPA) will help bind these toxins in the system for removal.

Once the heavy metals, pesticides or other chemicals have been bound to fats, the toxic fats are taken to the liver where they are eliminated by dumping them into the small intestines through the bile. Fiber is needed to bind these fats and heavy metals so they will be carried out of the body. While any kind of fiber helps, a particular form of mucilage known as sodium alginate is especially good at binding heavy metals.

These toxin-laden fats can also be eliminated through the skin. A close friend developed a rash on her hands after having amalgam fillings removed. The rash had a metallic taste to it, so we did some drawing baths with clay (See Chapter Nine) and a round of Heavy Metal Detox and it cleared up. Later, I had a similar rash on my feet after some dental work and the same program cleared it up for me.

Oral Chelation and Other Nutrients

The oral chelation program, discussed in the last chapter, is also very good at helping to eliminate heavy metals from the body. However, one doesn't have to do the full oral chelation program for MegaChel to act as a heavy metal cleanser. Just 1-2 tablets twice daily will help.

There are other nutrients that aid in eliminating heavy metals. Antioxidants like vitamin C and vitamin E are helpful. B-Complex vitamins can be useful in heavy metal detoxification. Several minerals also help the process, including magnesium, calcium, sulfur, selenium, and zinc. Many of these nutrients aid the enzyme systems involved in detoxification. Sulfur-rich foods like garlic and onions and cruciferous vegetables like broccoli and cabbage are very helpful in activating detoxification pathways. Indole-3 Carbinol is a constituent of cruciferous vegetables that aids in detoxification, especially when used with vitamin C.

Heavy Metal Cleanse

If you know or suspect you have heavy metal poisoning it's probably a good idea to work with an experienced doctor, naturopath or herbalist to custom design a program for your individual needs. However, as a starting point, here's a mercury and heavy metal detox program I've used on myself and others:

- 1 Tablespoon of Flax Seed oil twice daily
- 1 Heavy Metal Detox twice daily

- 2-4 Algin three times daily or 1 Tablespoon Nature's Three in a glass of water or juice twice daily

- Once or twice each week take a drawing bath with Hydrated Bentonite or another fine clay (see page 69)

Make certain the bowels are moving at least two to three times per day. If not, you may wish to take some LBS II at bedtime or 2 Magnesium Complex twice daily

- Optional: For a stronger effect add 1-2 MegaChel twice daily

Heavy metal detoxification is important for anyone who has worked around a lot of chemicals in their job (including painters beauticians, lab technicians, dry cleaners, carpet cleaners, farmers and factory workers in many industries). It's also a good thing for people suffering from any kind of chronic inflammatory disorder or problem that involves nerve damage.

Like tissue cleansing it's usually a good idea to do a general cleanse first to ensure the eliminative channels are open. Otherwise, the tissues dump heavy metals and the body can't eliminate them. If one develops a strong cleansing reaction to this program (as described above), it's best to stop or slow down and focus on some general cleansing procedures for a few days. Then resume the cleanse at a slower place. It's also wise to do what we can to avoid heavy metals and other toxins in the first place, which is the topic of our next chapter.

Chapter Fifteen

Protecting Ourselves in a Toxic World

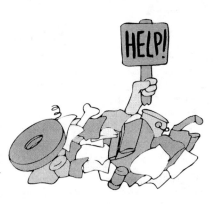

The phrase "environmental pollution" conjures up all sorts of images, like the sooty skyscraper chimneys belching out clouds of smoke that billow skyward, polluted lakes and streams, and toxic waste dumps.

It's not a pretty picture, but it is a common one throughout the world, especially third world and former communist nations. Just two decades ago it was very common in the United States. Things are improving thanks to public awareness of the problem, but in spite of great strides, there is still a long way to go. It's a problem we all need to be concerned about for the sake of our own health and well-being as well as future generations.

The point is, we are facing health challenges that no other people who have lived on the earth have ever faced before. Hence, we all need to be active in doing what we can to help clean up the pollution on our planet. However, our health and well-being also demand that we pay serious attention to protecting our own bodies against the threats of environmental pollution.

To combat environmental pollution (regardless of its sources) requires a strong immune system and a clean blood stream. So, start by cleaning up the internal environment of your own body by doing some cleansing as described in this book. But, doesn't it make more sense to keep toxins out of the body in the first place?

Since we live in a toxic environment, it is impossible to completely avoid toxic chemicals, but we should do as much as possible to minimize our exposure to them. Don't get paranoid about this, however. Remember, the body can handle a certain amount of toxicity, especially when provided with good nutrition and healthy attitudes.

Here are some specific ways you can minimize your exposure to environmental toxins.

Clean Up Your Water

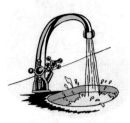

Next to air, water is the most important "nutrient" our body needs. Water is one of the greatest cleansers of the body, yet, ironically, it has become a major source of toxic exposure.

Tap water in most parts of the country is now laced with chemicals as a result of industrial contamination and agricultural runoff. Even where this is not a problem, the addition of chlorine to drinking water is a problem. While chlorination of water supplies has helped to prevent the spread of contagious diseases, the chlorine in our drinking water has introduced new health problems.

When chlorine combines with organic matter in the water it forms carcinogenic chemicals such as trihalomethanes and chloroform. Chlorine itself is a free radical and causes free radical damage. It changes HDL cholesterol (the good kind of cholesterol) into LDL cholesterol.

In fact, research done by Dr. Joseph Price discovered that the sudden rise in cardiovascular disease in the early 20th century directly paralleled the chlorination of water supplies. He performed laboratory research that demonstrated a high fat diet would not cause arteriosclerosis in laboratory animals if the animals were not given chlorinated water. Dr. Price wrote a book about his research entitled *Coronaries, Cholesterol and Chlorine*, which, unfortunately, is no longer in print.

Although Dr. Price was persecuted for his discoveries, his findings are vitally important to the health of every person on this planet. Heart disease is the number one cause of death in civilized countries, and Dr. Price's research shows this is directly linked to chlorine.

Chlorine is gradually being replaced with other chemicals in many municipal water supplies. One of these chemicals is bromine. Another common drinking water additive is fluoride. The evidence that fluoride prevents tooth decay is weak. The element fluorine, found in foods, is a valuable nutrient, but the fluoride added to drinking water is a toxic by-product of aluminum manufacturing. It is an endocrine disrupter for males, interfering with testosterone. It is also linked to increased cancer risk.

Chlorine, bromine and fluoride are all in the same column as iodine on the periodic table of elements. So, one of the other problems these chemicals pose is that they displace iodine in the body, which may be contributing to the extremely high rate of thyroid problems people are experiencing.

Again, these are just two of literally hundreds of chemicals that are finding their way into our water supply. Many people are recognizing they need pure water to be healthy, but what is the best way to obtain pure water?

Buying bottled water isn't necessarily the answer, because there are no quality standards for bottled water. However, it's good to find some quality brands you can use when traveling. For home use, bottled water is too expensive. Carbon filters are also unreliable for removing many contaminants from water. The two best methods are distillation and reverse osmosis, although there are other technologies for water purification that are emerging. Both reverse osmosis and distillation should be followed by carbon filtration for maximum effectiveness.

Nature's Spring

I use a Nature's Spring Reverse Osmosis unit to purify my drinking water at the tap. It has been one of the best investments in my health I've ever made. The water tastes great, too, which helps you drink more of it.

Nature's Spring utilizes a three-step water purification system. The first step in the water's journey to being cleaned is its passage through a five-micron pre-filter called a 'sock.' This filter removes the large particles and oxides, such as iron and suspended calcium, from the water. Any sediment that is in the water is also removed by the pre-filter. This pre-filter actually blocks many microbes, too.

The next step the water goes through is the reverse osmosis membrane that is the heart of the Nature's Spring unit. The filtration at this point involves a special membrane filter with such tiny pores that only select molecules, primarily oxygen and water, can pass through. One of the reasons water purified in this manner tastes so good is that the reverse osmosis process actually oxygenates the water, giving it a fresh, clean taste.

It works this way. As the water enters the reverse osmosis (R.O.) chamber it is forced against the membrane. That force creates just enough pressure to allow only small water molecule chains to pass through, all cleaned and purified. The undesirable part of the water is not able to pass through, so it deflects off the membrane and, with the waste water, takes a different pathway through a waste tube that dumps the waste water down the drain.

Reverse osmosis is a natural process. The sea gull uses an R.O. process in a membrane in its head to filter sea water. The Navy uses R.O. to purify its water supplies when out on long, ocean-going excursions. Some coastal communities are currently experimenting with reverse osmosis technology as an effective means of converting the abundance of salty sea water to potable drinking water for community use.

The final step in the water's journey to purification is the post filter. This is an activated charcoal filter that removes residual chlorine or gasses that pass through the membrane. It also helps to remove any odors or bad taste.

Reverse osmosis is less expensive than distillation and produces better tasting water. In fact, any families discover that having this clean, oxygenated water causes them to drink more water, thus improving the health of the kidneys, skin, digestive tract, blood and sweat glands. You may be pleasantly surprised at how this one simple change can improve your health.

Xenoestrogens

It was discovered over 50 years ago that certain chemicals were having a negative impact on the reproductive capability of wild animals. In spite of this, our society has continued to accept and use these chemicals because they offer "quick fixes" in modern agriculture. Some of these chemicals have now been dubbed "xenoestrogens".

Xenoestrogens are chemical compounds from environmental pollutants that bond to estrogen receptor sites. The term estrogen does not refer to a specific hormone. An estrogen is any natural or artificial substance that induces estrus (female fertility and desire to mate). The human body makes three different estrogens—estriol, estrone, and estrodial. "Xeno" is a Greek word meaning "foreigner, stranger or alien". So xenoestrogens are foreign or alien estrogens.

Xenoestrogens bond to receptor sites within cells to make specific changes in cellular activity. These chemical estrogens can disrupt the function of the endocrine system in two ways. First, they can mimic natural hormones and turn on cellular processes at the wrong time, or simply over-stimulate them. A second way they can disrupt the body's hormonal processes is to bond to receptor sites without stimulating them, blocking normal hormonal processes.

The results of this bonding can be cellular damage, the inappropriate activation of genes, or the disruption of normal hormonal processes.

Although these chemicals have been tested for safety, they have all been tested individually, not collectively. One experiment showed that, when 10 commonly encountered chemicals were mixed at a tenth of their individually active dose, the potency (measured as cell proliferation) was 10 times higher than expected. So, the synergistic effect of these chemicals is dangerous.

Furthermore, they do not readily degrade nor break down in the environment. In fact, they tend to accumulate in the fatty tissues of animals and become more concentrated the higher up the food chain you go. This may be one of the reasons that vegetarians have a lower incidence of breast cancer than meat eaters.

Chemicals that appear to have serious reproductive and endocrine disruptive effects include:

- Pesticides (2,4-D, DDT and many others)
- Organochlorides (dioxin, PPBs, PCBs and others)
- Heavy metals (cadmium, lead and mercury)
- Plastic ingredients

119

Health Hazards of Xenoestrogens

Xenoestrogens have been documented in causes of reproductive dysfunction and mutations in wild birds, frogs, reptiles and even mammals. However, the first species of animals to be affected were birds of prey, because they sit at the top of their food chain. The problems these chemicals have caused in wild animals should have "clued us in" to the harm they are causing human beings, but commercial interests have continued to push for their use.

Some of the possible effects these xenoestrogens are having on human beings include:

1. Earlier onset of puberty in young girls. Girls are entering puberty at younger and younger ages.

2. Increases in breast and prostate cancer. These tissues contain estrogen receptor sites and are extremely prone to genetic damage and the stimulation of excess growth by xenoestrogens. Other cancers of the reproductive organs may also be caused by xenoestrogens.

3. Uterine fibroids and other reproductive disorders in women. By overstimulating uterine tissue, excessive tissue growth is encouraged.

4. A world-wide decrease in male fertility.

5. An increase in obesity because they are stored in fat when the body can't eliminate them.

The problem of xenoestrogens is compounded by the fact that farmers are routinely adding hormones to animal feed to increase production of milk and eggs. These hormones are also finding their way into our food and causing glandular imbalances.

Both men and women need to become keenly aware of xenoestrogens, avoiding them as much as they possibly can. Organic fruits and vegetables should be purchased whenever available, and produce should be washed in a natural soap like Sunshine Concentrate, or some other natural soap to remove pesticide residues. Use only organic meat, dairy and eggs. Use glass or paper cartons instead of plastic containers whenever possible.

Another strategy to minimize exposure to xenoestrogens is to use natural plant-based estrogens to tie up estrogen receptor sites. Phytoestrogens are chemicals in plants that also bond to estrogen receptor sites. However, phytoestrogens have a much weaker estrogenic effect than natural estrogens or xenoestrogens. The theory is that by consuming foods rich in phytoestrogens, receptor sites will be tied up, resulting in less estrogen stimulation.

Soy products and other legumes (beans and peas) are rich in phytoestrogens. Other sources include dark green vegetables and whole grains. Herbal sources include red clover, licorice, black cohosh and hops. PhytoSoy and Breast Assured are helpful supplements.

Food Additives

The average American consumes several pounds of food additives each year. These include artificial colorings and flavorings, preservatives, artificial sweeteners, flavor enhancers and many more. The liver has to process all of these chemicals as foreign substances, which places a great deal of stress on that organ. We should do our best to avoid food additives in general, but there are two food additives I'd like to call particular attention to—MSG and aspartame.

MSG, short for monosodium glutamate, is a flavor enhancer additive from the orient. Headaches, arthritic symptoms, malaise, and digestive distress are some of the symptoms caused by reactions to MSG. These symptoms have sometimes been called "Chinese restaurant syndrome" because of the liberal use of MSG in Chinese foods. Most prepackaged foods, especially soups, contain MSG! MSG should always be avoided.

Many people who are trying to make healthy lifestyle and diet changes have switched to aspartame in order to avoid refined sugar. However, it makes little sense to put an artificially synthesized chemical into the body, hoping to make healthful changes.

Marketed under the names Nutrasweet® and Equal®, aspartame has the same calorie content per gram as sugar but is about 200 times sweeter. Aspartame's sweetness is the most common reason for its use in calorie-reduced foods, although researchers have found aspartame to be ineffective in weight loss programs overall.

At first glance, the elements found in this sugar substitute seem harmless. Aspartame is made of two amino acids, phenylalanine and aspartic acid. But phenylalanine is toxic to individuals afflicted with the advanced liver disease, phenylketonuria (PKU), and high blood levels of phenylalanine during pregnancy (which subjects the fetus to poisonous levels of phenylalanine).

Similarly, aspartic acid is linked with the destruction of brain cells, according to some scientific studies. However, methyl (wood) alcohol, another substance found in aspartame, raises the most cause for alarm since methyl alcohol is converted within the body to formaldehyde and formic acid, both harmful poisons. These chemicals are highly toxic to the thymus gland, which produces T-lymphocytes for immune defense.

Aspartame's toxic ingredients may explain its link to such health problems as nausea, recurrent headaches, seizures, rashes, blindness, and brain damage. Additionally, this sweetener has been found to interfere with the body's neurotransmitters, which can lead to behavioral changes including moodiness, hallucinations, twitching, abnormal breathing and depression. Aspartame should be carefully avoided. Read labels!

These are just two of the many additives found in our food supply. We should avoid them all as much as possible. The solution is simple. Buy whole, natural foods instead of prepared foods as much as possible. Again, read labels. You don't need to know what all the additives are, just follow a simple rule—if you can't pronounce it, you probably shouldn't be eating it.

Household Chemicals

Our homes are filled with chemical substances in laundry detergents, soaps, chemical disinfectants, antiseptic hand cleaners, toothpaste, cosmetics and deodorants. Space does not permit an in-depth discussion of some of the potentially harmful chemicals in these products. Wherever possible, use more natural alternatives for these products.

Use natural, biodegradable cleaning products. Sunshine Concentrate and Nature's Fresh make excellent household cleaning products. Essential oils make great natural disinfectants.

Another source of chemicals is indoor pollution. Formaldehyde, the substance used to preserve dead bodies, is now routinely added to commercial building materials. Add to this the solvents found in paint, calk, adhesives and glues, plus the chemicals added to make carpets and upholstery stain resistant and you have a lot of chemical substances being released into the air in any new home. This is why many people feel sick or get headaches after remodeling or moving into a new home. This problem has been dubbed "indoor pollution".

Besides allowing for adequate ventilation, there is an easy way to deal with the problem of indoor pollution—houseplants. Plants help clear toxic chemicals out of the air. So, air out your home as often as is practical, and keep some houseplants to clean up the environment.

Tampering with Our Food Supply

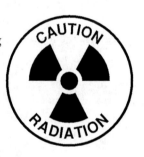

There are many other substances finding their way into our environment and food supply. In many cases, the long term effects of these substances are unknown. Two of the latest controversies are irradiation of foods and genetically-modified organisms (GMOs).

Although irradiation of foods does not make foods radioactive, it does alter them molecularly. Even microwaving foods alters the molecular structure of foods.

Many years ago, I read a report in *FDA Consumer* warning the public not to warm breast milk in a microwave oven because infants fed microwaved milk failed to thrive. This does not surprise me as microwaving would destroy enzymes and molecularly alter nutrient structures.

Some friends of mine did a little study to prove that I was wrong about the harmful effects of their microwave oven. They grew some sprouts in two different kinds of water—water that had been boiled on the stove top and water that had been boiled in a microwave. To their surprise, the seeds sprouted in the microwaved water took longer to sprout, had a lower germination rate, and spoiled faster. Needless to say, they stopped using their microwave.

Later, another friend had her daughter repeat the above experiment for a science fair project with similar results. It appears that microwaves alter the molecular structure of the water, and if it's bad for the health of plants, it's probably bad for us.

If microwaves can do this to the food, how much more damage is done when food is irradiated? As a result, I avoid irradiated foods, and I don't use a microwave oven, ever!

GMOs, which have been humorously referred to as frankenfoods, are another big threat to our health. As we tamper with the genetic structure of our food crops, who knows what the long-term results will be? The simple fact is, we don't know. Yet, in spite of the poor track record of the safety of our technologies on our own health and the environment, we continue to race ahead without considering the long-term consequences of our actions.

Native Americans were taught to consider the consequences of their choices on future generations. We need to start thinking about how our actions will affect our grandchildren seven generations into the future, instead of thinking about how they will affect quarterly corporate profits.

Hopefully, as more and more people wake up to the problem, the demand for safer, less toxic products and more natural foods and household products will increase. For now, the best way to initiate change is to vote with our dollars. My purchase decisions are influenced by my concern for the future of my great grandchildren, and my own health has improved as a result of those choices.

Chapter Sixteen

Letting Go of It

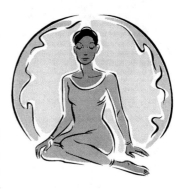

Detoxifying our bodies and avoiding environmental toxins are important health issues for the 21st century. However, in some ways, they are metaphors for an even more important health issue. More and more research is suggesting that what we are experiencing in the world around us is a result of consciousness—that is, our outer world is a projection of our inner world. If this is true, the growing toxicity in our physical world suggests a growing toxicity in our inner mental and emotional worlds.

Anger, hatred, resentment, greed, and other emotional states based in fear and negativity are just as toxic to us as pesticides, xenoestrogens and heavy metals. In fact, they are worse it some ways because they poison our very being, not just the physical body we inhabit. These are the toxins that don't enter the body from the outside; they are the toxins that defile us from within—the ones that arise from the heart.

Unfortunately, many of us seek to deal with these mental and emotional toxins in the same way we try to deal with physical toxins. We ignore the problem and seek to suppress the symptoms. We have to find a way to allow these emotions to surface and pass out of us. This is done, not by denying them, but by confronting them, acknowledging them and allowing them to wash through us and out of us.

Just stuffing these emotions inside and pretending they don't exist is equivalent to suppressing the eliminative functions of the body with drugs. Our tissues simply store the trauma. We develop emotional cysts and tumors, and become weighed down by accumulated emotional baggage. Typically, the excess physical weight we carry and the chronic health problems we experience have as much to do with our mental, emotional and spiritual toxicity as they do with our physical toxicity.

To solve any problem, we first must become aware of it, and often the physical symptoms we experience are trying to wake us up to the fact that "something is wrong." We need to realize that sickness often provides us with a much-needed opportunity for self-reflection—an opportunity to see the truth of what is really inside us.

We spend a lot of time and energy trying to stuff down feelings of fear, anger or pain that we don't want to acknowledge. We also focus the energy of these emotions outward in blame. We create a story that allows us to place the responsibility for how we feel on other people and we tell the story of our "victimization" over and over again to justify our inner emotional experience. However, the stories we tell aren't who we really are, and since we "wrote" them in the first place, we have the capacity to "rewrite" them, and release the burdens we are carrying in the process.

How do we do this? Well, start by watching your thoughts. Your thoughts aren't who you really are, they are just "programs" that are running in your physical brain. Many are programs you didn't even write. They were written by parents, teachers, siblings and others when you were young. You have the capacity to "let go" of negative thought patterns and replace them with positive ones.

Affirmations

One of the methods of doing this is to use positive affirmations. An affirmation is a present tense statement that affirms what one wants as if one currently possessed it. I've used this tool many times in my own life. I changed my attitudes about money from the "poverty mentality" I inherited from my parents to a belief that "God provides for my every need and good desire," through affirmations.

Notice that the affirmation is a present tense statement. This is a vital secret to making affirmations work because it is laying hold of what is desired in the present tense. If a person says, "Someday I will have all the money I need," someday never comes. They are placing the time of change in the future, not the present. The power to let go of old thoughts and habits and change them into new positive ones is in the present, not in the future.

I often suggest affirmations that clients can repeat to themselves in order to crowd out negative thoughts and emotions. Where there is a particularly difficult issue, it can help to phrase the affirmation as a question, "What would it feel like if..." So, if a person is depressed and unhappy, they might ask themselves repeatedly, "What would it feel like to be motivated and happy?" The only way the body can answer such a question is to start generating the feeling of being motivated and happy, so this technique can be a very powerful one for helping a person to change their attitudes and feelings.

However, positive thinking isn't enough. We also need to start saying "yes" to how we feel instead of "no." When we feel pain, hurt, sadness, anger, fear, etc. we start by acknowledging it. Instead of saying, "You hurt me" or "He made me angry," we simply own the feeling. We say, "Yes, I am feeling hurt" or "Yes, I am feeling angry." Owning something is the first step to being able to let it go.

Breathing

Usually, when we start feeling something we don't want to feel we hold our breath. This suppresses the body's energy and numbs our ability to feel. It also shuts off our lymphatic system and causes our tissues to hold onto toxicity. Seen from this perspective, holding our breath is one of the primary ways we become toxic, both physically and emotionally.

The key is to acknowledge the feeling and then keep breathing. When we breathe through a feeling instead of trying to make it go away, it finds a way to "vent" and escape. We may cry, yell, hit a pillow, or otherwise "act out" the feeling, but as long as we aren't harming ourselves or other people there is nothing wrong with this. If you breathe through it, the sensation will pass and the emotional toxin will escape, just like physical toxins will be eliminated as the body gets stronger.

Physical health is a state of balance, characterized by a high level of energy and a sense of well-being. Feelings of inner peace, love and calm are the healthy state of our being. These are the states of being our innermost self is craving and deviations from this state are signs that we need to detoxify our inner being.

What fiber, water and herbs do for the physical body, acknowledgement, breathing and forgiveness will do for our spirit. Forgiveness is the ultimate act of cleansing. It is letting go of the blame, guilt and judgments we have of other people. It is the release of emotional toxins that cleanses the heart and allows nourishing peace, love and joy to nourish our soul.

So, in the process of cleansing the body, don't forget to cleanse your being. As you acknowledge feelings and hurt, sadness, anger, fear, worry, blame, guilt, etc., breathe through them. As you breathe, exhale fully and say, "I release this feeling" or "I forgive this person completely." Exhaling is the way we "let go" of things, so push all the air out of your lungs and imagine that you are exhaling all of the pain out of your body as you do so.

When you forgive, release and "let go," you will feel lighter, both physically and emotionally. Feelings of hurt and pain will be replaced with feelings of peace and joy as you inhale fully after your emptying out is finished. Learn to "let go of it" and you will experience renewed health and vitality on every level, not just the physical plane. Start "Coming Clean" today.

For more information on cleansing, physically and emotionally, see the *Suggested Additional Reading* materials on the next page.

Additional Reading

On Detoxification and Physical Cleansing

Colon Cleansing: The Best-Kept Secret by Jennifer Weiss and Vena Burnett

Detoxification by Linda R. Page

Food is Your Best Medicine by Henry Bieler

Guess What Came to Dinner?: Parasites and Your Health by Ann Louise Gittleman, Omar M. Amin

Is Any Sick Among You? by LaDean Griffin

Rational Fasting by Arnold Ehret

Sweet Poison: How The World's Most Popular Artificial Sweetener Is Killing Us by Janet Starr Hull

The '90s Healthy Body Book: How to Overcome the Effects of Pollution and Cleanse the Toxins from Your Body by Gary Null

The Colon Health Handbook by Robert Gray

The Cure for All Diseases by Hulda Regehr Clark

The Detox Diet: A How-To & When-To Guide for Cleansing the Body by Elson M. Haas

The Foundations of Health: The Liver and Digestive Herbal by Christopher Hobbs

The Master Cleanser by Stanley Burroughs

The Mucusless Diet Healing System by Arnold Ehret

The Yeast Connection by William G. Crook

Why Suffer? by Ann Wigmore

On Mental and Emotional Cleansing

"CLEAR" – Tree of Light Course by Kimberly Balas and Laura McCready

"Emotional Anatomy" – Tree of Light Course by Steven Horne

Feelings Buried Alive Never Die by Karol Kuhn Truman

Flower Essence Repertory by Patricia Kaminski and Richard Katz

"Love Your Body Beautiful" Tree of Light Course by Deanna Hansen and Steven Horne

Seven Herbs: Plants as Teachers by Matthew Wood

The Body Has Its Reasons by Therese Bertherat and Carol Bernstein http://www.antigymnastique.com/anglais/tb.html

The Dragon Doesn't Live Here Anymore by Alan Cohen

The Language of the Body by Alexander Lown

For additional information and resources visit www.treelite.com.

Special Offers

Free Cleansing Resource CD

Thank you for purchasing this book. As our way of saying thank you, we'd like to offer you a free CD on cleansing which you can use for your own information, or to help others with the process of "Coming Clean." The CD features a short audio presentation by Steven Horne on the importance of cleansing and a series of handouts on cleansing products and programs which can be printed out to use for yourself, friends, family or clients.

This CD is available for a $4.50 shipping and handling charge. To get your free CD, photocopy this page, fill in the information below and mail it to: Tree of Light Publishing, P.O. Box 911239, St. George, UT 84791. You can also fax the form to 435-627-2367 or phone in the information by calling 800-416-2887. Only one free CD per customer. Additional CDs are $9.95 plus shipping.

— — — — — — — — — — — — —

Please send me my free Cleansing Resource CD

Name _____

Address _____

City, State and Zip _____

Phone _____ Email _____

_____ I have enclosed a check for $4.50 for shipping and handling.

_____ Please bill the credit card listed below for the $4.50 shipping and handling charge

Card Number _____

Expiration Date _____

Signature _____

Other Information on Cleansing

Tree of Light publishing offers the following materials which contain additional information on cleansing and other natural methods for improving your health.

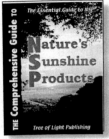

$29.95

The Comprehensive Guide to Nature's Sunshine Products

Featuring 633 NSP products available in the United States and Canada, this book provides a comprehensive list of properties, body system's affected, historical uses, directions for use, and warnings and contraindications for each product. It also provides charts and instructions for the ABC+D Approach to Natural Healing, and a therapuetic index to over 500 health problems.

Dr. Mom-Dr. Dad Course

For the price of only 1-2 doctor visits, this course helps people can rediscover the value of primary health care in the home by learning how to overcome many health problems in less time than it takes to get an appointment to see the doctor. In the Dr. Mom-Dr. Dad course, we explain how to relieve pain from minor injuries, how to help the body quickly recover from acute illnesses and how to build overall health to reduce the incidence of disease in your home, and reverse many chronic ailments. All of this can be accomplished with no drugs or medications, only safe, natural methods.

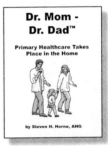

$124.98

The ABC+D Approach Course

The key to helping people with herbs, nutrition and other natural healing modalities is results. We've made learning to do this much easier, by creating the ABC+D Health Consulting System™. The ABC+D course teaches you how to help people modify their lifestyle to remove the root causes (using the principles of Active, Build and Cleanse) and by providing Direct Aid to balance biological terrain and support the function of the various body systems. The two videos and 137 page manual in this course enable one to start effectively consulting with people in a very short period of time.

$99.98

Visit our website at www.treelite.com or call 800-416-2887 for a free catalog

Additional copies of this book are
available through:

Tree of Light Publishing

www.treelite.com

800-416-2887